THE SCIENCE-BACKED GUIDE

TO

LIVE A PAIN-FREE LIFE

Evidence-Based Strategies for Chronic Pain Recovery
Through Neuroplasticity, Sleep, Nutrition & Mindfulness

BRIANNA BROWN

ISBN: 978-1-257-78593-3

Published by: Sharp Press

TABLE OF CONTENTS

INTRODUCTION

What if everything you've been told about chronic pain is wrong?

What if the shooting pain in your back, the persistent ache in your joints, or the relentless throb in your head isn't a life sentence but rather a challenge your brain has been trained to solve? What if the answer to your pain doesn't lie in another prescription, another injection, or another surgery, but in the remarkable, untapped healing power of your own mind and body working in harmony?

I'm not asking you to believe in miracles or abandon science. Quite the opposite. I'm asking you to embrace the most exciting scientific revolution in pain medicine—discoveries so profound they're rewriting medical textbooks and transforming lives around the world. This isn't false hope; it's evidence-based hope backed by hundreds of rigorous clinical studies and brain imaging research that proves what thousands of people are already experiencing: chronic pain can be dramatically reduced, and in many cases, completely eliminated.

The Pain Crisis That Demands a New Solution

Right now, as you read this, approximately 20% of adults worldwide—over 1.5 billion people—are living with chronic pain. In the United States alone, chronic pain affects more people than diabetes, heart disease, and cancer combined. The economic burden exceeds $635 billion annually, but the human cost is incalculable: destroyed careers, shattered relationships, lost dreams, and lives lived in the shadow of suffering.

For decades, our medical system has responded to this crisis with increasingly powerful medications, more invasive procedures, and treatments that often fail to address the root causes of persistent pain. We've created a generation of pain patients who've been told their conditions are permanent, their pain is "just something they'll have to live with," and their best hope is to "manage" their suffering rather than eliminate it.

But here's the truth that's emerging from research laboratories around the globe: the brain "creates" pain, but it also has the capacity to reduce or even eliminate it. The significance of this discovery cannot be overstated. If your brain constructs your pain experience—and mounting evidence proves it does—then your brain can also deconstruct it.

The Scientific Revolution Changing Everything

In laboratories at Harvard, Stanford, Oxford, and research centers worldwide, neuroscientists are uncovering mechanisms that would have seemed like science fiction just a decade ago. Recent studies show that chronic pain involves changes in the central nervous system, including mechanisms like central sensitization and neuroplasticity. These aren't just technical terms—they represent the keys to your freedom.

Consider these groundbreaking findings from 2024 and 2025 research:

The Brain's Pain Construction System: Advanced brain imaging reveals that the spontaneous pain of chronic back pain engages brain regions that modulate emotional evaluation relative to the self, not just sensory pain areas. Your pain isn't just happening *to* you—your brain is actively creating it based on emotions, memories, expectations, and beliefs.

The Sleep-Pain Revolution: Emerging evidence suggests that the effect of sleep on pain may be even stronger than the effect of pain on sleep. This means that by mastering your sleep, you can dramatically reduce your pain—often more effectively than with medications.

Mindfulness as Medicine: Mindfulness-based pain management (MBPM) has evidenced significant positive changes in patients with chronic pain, with clinical trials showing it can outperform traditional treatments for many conditions.

Nutrition as Pain Medicine: Recent research demonstrates that adopting a healthy diet can reduce the severity of chronic pain, presenting an easy and accessible way for sufferers to better manage their condition—independent of body weight.

Movement as Healing: Yoga has been proven to be an effective therapy for chronic low back pain, with studies showing it can be as effective as physical therapy and superior to standard medical care.

Beyond Band-Aid Solutions

This book isn't about managing your pain—it's about eliminating it. We're moving beyond the outdated model that treats symptoms while ignoring causes. Instead, you'll discover how to address the neurobiological, psychological, physical, and social factors that create and maintain chronic pain.

The approaches you'll learn aren't experimental or unproven. They're backed by rigorous research, including randomized controlled trials, systematic reviews, and meta-analyses published in the world's most prestigious medical journals. Every technique, every strategy, every protocol in this book has been tested in real-world clinical settings with real people suffering from real pain.

What Makes This Guide Different

Unlike other pain books that focus on single solutions, this guide integrates the full spectrum of evidence-based approaches into a comprehensive system. You'll discover how neuroplasticity training, mindfulness-based pain management, sleep optimization, anti-inflammatory nutrition, therapeutic movement, and social connection work synergistically to create lasting pain relief.

But more importantly, you'll learn how to personalize these approaches for your unique situation. Chronic pain affects everyone differently, influenced by genetics, life experiences, stress levels, sleep patterns, social support, and dozens of other factors. This isn't a one-size-fits-all program—it's a sophisticated toolkit that adapts to your individual needs.

The Journey Ahead

Over the next ten chapters, you'll embark on a journey of discovery that will fundamentally change your relationship with pain. You'll learn to see your pain not as an enemy to fight, but as a sophisticated alarm system that can be reprogrammed. You'll discover that your brain—the same organ that may have trapped you in chronic pain— also holds the master key to your freedom.

Chapter by chapter, you'll build a comprehensive understanding of how pain works and, more importantly, how healing happens. You'll develop practical skills you can use immediately while building toward long-term transformation. By the time you finish this book, you won't just understand the science of pain relief—you'll be living it.

A Promise Based on Science

I won't promise you'll be pain-free overnight. Transformation takes time, especially when you're rewiring neural pathways that may have been entrenched for years. But I will promise you this: if you apply the evidence-based approaches in this book consistently and patiently, you will experience significant improvement in your pain levels, your function, and your quality of life.

This promise isn't based on hope or wishful thinking. It's based on the accumulated evidence of thousands of clinical studies and the real-world experiences of people who've walked this path before you. The relationship between nutrition and chronic pain is complex and may involve many underlying mechanisms such as oxidative stress, inflammation, and glucose metabolism, requiring a comprehensive and interdisciplinary approach that includes nutrition—and every other aspect of your life.

Your Pain-Free Future Starts Now

The age of accepting chronic pain as permanent is ending. The age of true, science-based healing is beginning. Your brain has spent months, years, or even decades perfecting the art of pain creation. Now it's time to teach it the art of pain elimination.

Are you ready to discover what your body has been trying to tell you? Are you prepared to unlock the healing power that's been within you all along? Are you willing to embrace the possibility that your pain-free future isn't just a dream, but a scientifically-supported reality waiting to unfold?

If so, turn the page. Your transformation begins now.

Welcome to the future of pain medicine. Welcome to your pain-free life.

CHAPTER 1: THE PAIN PARADOX

Imagine if I told you that the most sophisticated pain relief system ever created already exists—and it's sitting right between your ears. For centuries, we've been looking in all the wrong places for pain relief: in pills, procedures, and surgeries. But the most groundbreaking discovery in modern pain science reveals a startling truth that flips everything we thought we knew on its head: your brain doesn't just receive pain signals, it actively constructs your entire pain experience.

This isn't just an interesting scientific curiosity—it's the key to your freedom. Because if your brain creates pain, it can also eliminate it. Recent advances in neuroscience have revealed that chronic pain is influenced by changes in the central nervous system, including mechanisms like central sensitization and neuroplasticity. This means that the very organ responsible for your suffering also holds the master blueprint for your healing.

The implications are staggering. We're not talking about simply managing pain or learning to cope better—we're talking about the possibility of complete elimination of chronic pain through scientifically proven methods that work with your brain's natural healing mechanisms.

Breaking Down the Construction Zone in Your Head

Traditional medicine has operated under what researchers call the "nociceptive model"—the idea that pain works like a sophisticated alarm system. According to this outdated view, when tissue is damaged, specialized pain receptors called nociceptors send danger signals up your spinal cord to your brain, which then creates pain proportional to the damage. More tissue damage equals more pain, and pain should disappear when tissues heal.

But here's where this model completely breaks down, and where the pain paradox reveals itself: extensive research now shows that pain has very little correlation with actual tissue damage. Studies consistently demonstrate that people can have significant structural abnormalities—herniated discs, arthritis, torn cartilage—yet experience no pain whatsoever. Conversely, people can experience excruciating chronic pain with little to no detectable tissue damage.

The brain "creates" pain, but it also has the capacity to reduce or even eliminate it. This revolutionary understanding emerged from decades of brain imaging studies that revealed something extraordinary: the spontaneous pain of chronic back pain engages mPFC, a brain region that modulates emotional evaluation relative to the self. Your pain isn't just a simple sensory experience—it's a complex construction project involving memory, emotion, expectation, attention, and social context.

Think of your brain as an incredibly sophisticated computer running multiple programs simultaneously. The "pain program" integrates information from dozens of sources: sensory input from your body, memories of past pain experiences, current stress levels, sleep quality, emotional state, beliefs about your condition, social support, and even cultural factors about how pain should be expressed and experienced. Based on all this information, your brain makes a split-second decision: "How much pain should this person experience right now?"

The Central Sensitization Revolution

One of the most important breakthroughs in understanding chronic pain involves a phenomenon called central sensitization. Chronic neuropathic pain is a debilitating neuroplastic disorder that notably impacts the quality of life of millions of people worldwide. This complex condition, encompassing various manifestations, such as sciatica, diabetic neuropathy and postherpetic neuralgia, arises from nerve damage or malfunctions in pain processing pathways and involves various biological, physiological and psychological processes. Maladaptive neuroplasticity, known as central sensitization, plays a critical role in the persistence of chronic neuropathic pain.

Central sensitization occurs when your nervous system gets stuck in a hypersensitive state, like a car alarm that goes off when someone walks by, not just when someone tries to break in. These regions exhibit gray matter decrease and changes in connectivity during chronic pain. Several cortical networks, mainly the central executive network, the default mode network, and the salience network exhibit neuroplasticity which reallocates cognitive and emotional resources to pain processing.

What makes central sensitization so problematic—and so hopeful— is that it represents pure neuroplasticity in action. Your nervous system has literally rewired itself to prioritize danger signals and amplify pain responses. The pathways that were supposed to protect you have become oversensitive, firing pain signals in response to normal, harmless sensations.

But here's the paradox that offers hope: if your nervous system can change in ways that increase pain, it can also change in ways that decrease pain. Neuroplasticity refers to the capacity for variation and adaptive alterations in the morphology and functionality of neurons and synapses, and it plays a significant role in the transmission and modulation of pain. The same mechanisms that created your chronic pain can be harnessed to eliminate it.

Why Tissue Damage Doesn't Predict Your Pain Experience

The disconnect between tissue damage and pain intensity isn't just an interesting scientific observation—it's a fundamental truth that liberates millions of people from the fear that their pain means ongoing harm. Research consistently shows that structural abnormalities on medical imaging often have little relationship to pain levels.

Consider the research on back pain, one of the most common chronic pain conditions. Studies of people with no back pain whatsoever reveal that approximately 30% of 20-year-olds, 60% of 50-year-olds, and 84% of 80-year-olds have disc degeneration visible on MRI scans. These "abnormalities" are often just normal signs of aging, like wrinkles on the inside.

Even more striking are studies of people who've had major tissue healing. We argued that this pattern of changes in brain morphometry may be related to the shift in CBP pain perception from sensory (nociceptive) to emotional (hedonic) areas of the brain. The chronic pain system has essentially hijacked brain regions responsible for emotional processing, meaning your pain experience becomes more about your brain's interpretation than your body's condition.

This revelation frees you from one of the most limiting beliefs in chronic pain: that pain equals damage. Your MRI findings, your X-rays, your diagnostic tests—while important for ruling out serious pathology—don't determine your pain experience or your potential for recovery. Your brain does.

The Neuroplasticity Advantage

Neuroplasticity—your brain's ability to reorganize and form new neural connections throughout your life—represents the biological foundation of hope for chronic pain sufferers. Neuroplasticity forms the basis for important functions such as learning and memory, but it is also a mechanism of neurological and psychiatric disorders, and structural and functional neuroplastic changes are observed in pain conditions.

For decades, scientists believed that adult brains were essentially fixed structures, unable to change significantly after a critical period in childhood. This limiting belief suggested that chronic pain, once established, was permanent. But revolutionary research over the past two decades has shattered this myth completely.

We now know that your brain changes constantly throughout your life in response to experience, learning, and focused practice. These interventions help rewire the brain's pain pathways, promoting long-term pain relief and functional recovery. Every time you learn something new, every time you practice a skill, every time you change a habit, you're literally rewiring your brain at the cellular level.

The implications for chronic pain are extraordinary. These techniques can alter neural activity without surgery, offering a safer alternative to traditional treatments. Research shows that specific, targeted interventions can promote beneficial neuroplastic changes that reduce pain, improve function, and restore quality of life.

Modern neuroscience has identified several key mechanisms through which beneficial neuroplasticity occurs in pain conditions:

Synaptic Plasticity: The strength of connections between neurons can be modified through experience and practice. Interventions like mindfulness meditation and cognitive training can strengthen connections in pain-inhibiting pathways while weakening connections in pain-amplifying circuits.

Structural Plasticity: Actual physical changes in brain anatomy, including the growth of new neurons and the formation of new neural pathways. Studies show that people who engage in neuroplasticity-based interventions develop measurable increases in gray matter volume in brain regions associated with pain modulation.

Functional Plasticity: Changes in how different brain regions communicate and coordinate their activity. Understanding these changes provides insight into the role of subcortical structures in chronic pain and their potential as therapeutic targets.

The Bidirectional Nature of Neuroplastic Change

One of the most important aspects of neuroplasticity in chronic pain is that it works in both directions. Just as maladaptive neuroplastic changes can increase pain sensitivity and maintain chronic pain, adaptive neuroplastic changes can decrease pain sensitivity and promote healing.

Maladaptive plasticity is linked to the chronification of diseases such as pain, but the transition from acute to chronic pain is not well understood mechanistically. Research reveals that the transition from acute to chronic pain involves specific neuroplastic changes in key brain regions, including the central nucleus of the amygdala, which plays a crucial role in both the sensory and emotional aspects of pain.

But this same research provides the roadmap for reversal. Neuroplasticity in the central nucleus of the amygdala (CeA) has emerged as a mechanism for sensory and emotional-affective aspects of injury-induced pain, and understanding these mechanisms allows us to develop interventions that promote healing-oriented neuroplastic changes.

Breaking Free from the Permanence Myth

Perhaps the most liberating aspect of understanding neuroplasticity in chronic pain is how it demolishes the myth of permanence. For too long, people with chronic pain have been told their conditions are progressive, degenerative, or permanent. They've been encouraged to "accept" their limitations and focus on "managing" rather than healing.

This defeatist approach isn't just psychologically damaging—it's scientifically inaccurate. We propose that understanding and manipulating processes underlying the emotional suffering (cortical-limbic circuitry) should be more successful in treating chronic pain, as compared to the standard approaches that have been tested for decades.

The research reveals that chronic pain is not a fixed state but a dynamic process that can be influenced, modified, and even reversed through appropriate interventions. We redefine chronic pain as pain that does not extinguish its memory trace. The latter definition assumes the critical role of mesocorticolimbic circuitry in the control of pain chronification.

This redefinition is crucial because it shifts focus from damaged tissues to maladaptive memory traces—and memories can be updated, modified, and even overwritten through targeted interventions.

The Integration Imperative

Understanding that your brain constructs your pain experience doesn't mean that physical factors don't matter or that pain is "all in your head." Rather, it reveals that effective pain treatment must address the full spectrum of factors that influence brain function: biological, psychological, social, and spiritual.

These methods take advantage of the brain's plasticity for healing, from virtual reality and brain-computer interfaces to constraint-induced movement therapy. Modern pain science shows us that the most effective approaches integrate multiple modalities that work synergistically to promote beneficial neuroplastic changes.

Your journey to pain freedom begins with this fundamental understanding: you are not at the mercy of damaged tissues, faulty genes, or permanent dysfunction. You have a brain capable of extraordinary change, healing, and adaptation. The same neuroplasticity that may have contributed to your chronic pain can be your greatest ally in eliminating it.

In the chapters that follow, you'll learn exactly how to harness this remarkable capacity for change through evidence-based interventions that promote healing-oriented neuroplasticity. Your pain-free future isn't just possible—given what we now know about the brain's capacity for change, it's the expected outcome when you apply the right approaches consistently and systematically.

The paradox of pain is also the promise of pain: the brain that creates your suffering also holds the key to your freedom.

CHAPTER 2: REWIRING YOUR PAIN PATHWAYS

Understanding Central Sensitization

Your nervous system operates like a sophisticated security system, constantly monitoring for threats and adjusting its sensitivity based on perceived danger levels. Under normal circumstances, this system works flawlessly—detecting genuine threats while filtering out harmless sensations. But in chronic pain conditions, something goes fundamentally wrong: the security system gets stuck in maximum alert mode, treating every sensation as a potential threat.

Central sensitization represents one of the most significant breakthroughs in understanding chronic pain mechanisms. Chronic neuropathic pain is a debilitating neuroplastic disorder that notably impacts the quality of life of millions of people worldwide. Maladaptive neuroplasticity, known as central sensitization, plays a critical role in the persistence of chronic neuropathic pain.

This process fundamentally alters how your nervous system processes sensory information. These regions exhibit gray matter decrease and changes in connectivity during chronic pain. Several cortical networks, mainly the central executive network, the default mode network, and the salience network exhibit neuroplasticity which reallocates cognitive and emotional resources to pain processing.

When central sensitization occurs, several critical changes happen simultaneously in your nervous system:

Hyperexcitability: Neurons become overly responsive to stimuli that would normally be ignored or processed as non-threatening. A gentle touch might register as burning pain. Light pressure becomes excruciating. Movement that should feel normal triggers alarm signals.

Expanded Receptive Fields: Pain neurons begin responding to stimuli from larger areas of the body than they should. What starts as localized pain spreads to regions that shouldn't be affected. This explains why chronic pain often expands beyond the original injury site.

Altered Threshold Responses: The threshold for triggering pain responses drops dramatically. Sensations that would normally require significant stimulation to register as pain now trigger intense responses with minimal input.

Temporal Summation: Repeated stimuli that individually wouldn't cause pain begin to build up and create intense pain responses. This "wind-up" phenomenon means that activities you could previously tolerate become impossible.

The revolutionary aspect of understanding central sensitization is recognizing that these changes represent neuroplasticity in action— your nervous system has learned to be hypersensitive. But because these changes are learned, they can also be unlearned through targeted interventions that promote adaptive neuroplastic changes.

The Neuroplasticity Training Revolution

Modern neuroscience has identified specific protocols that can systematically retrain your nervous system to process sensory information normally again. Pain Neuroscience Education (PNE), mindfulness practices, and cognitive functional therapy (CFT), which target these neurobiological changes to improve pain perception and behaviors. These interventions help rewire the brain's pain pathways, promoting long-term pain relief and functional recovery.

Pain Neuroscience Education (PNE)

Pain Neuroscience Education represents a fundamental shift from traditional pain education approaches. Rather than focusing on anatomical structures or biomechanical explanations, PNE teaches patients about the neuroscience of pain processing itself. Key educational topics in PNE include the biopsychosocial model of pain, the concept of central sensitization, the relationship between pain and tissue damage, and the neuroplasticity of the nervous system.

Research demonstrates PNE's effectiveness across multiple chronic pain conditions. Recent studies have demonstrated PNE's effectiveness across various chronic pain conditions, such as chronic low back pain, fibromyalgia, and chronic widespread pain. The educational process employs tools like visual metaphors, real-life examples, and interactive explanations to enhance patient comprehension and engagement.

PNE works by fundamentally changing how your brain interprets sensory signals. When you understand that pain is constructed in your brain rather than simply transmitted from damaged tissues, several important cognitive shifts occur:

Reconceptualization of Pain: Understanding that pain doesn't always equal damage reduces fear and catastrophic thinking associated with pain sensations.

Increased Self-Efficacy: Knowledge about neuroplasticity and the brain's capacity for change increases confidence in your ability to influence your pain experience.

Reduced Fear-Avoidance: Understanding the difference between hurt and harm allows for gradual return to normal activities without the fear that movement will cause additional damage.

Enhanced Treatment Engagement: Knowing how different interventions work at the neurobiological level increases motivation and adherence to treatment protocols.

Mindfulness-Based Neuroplasticity Training

Mindfulness practices represent one of the most well-researched neuroplasticity training approaches for chronic pain. Accruing evidence supports the clinical efficacy of mindfulness treatments in reducing chronic pain symptoms. MBPM had enhancing effects on cognitive performance related to attention, inhibitory control, and psychological well-being.

The neurobiological mechanisms underlying mindfulness-based pain relief involve multiple systems:

Attention Regulation: Mindfulness training strengthens prefrontal cortex regions responsible for attention control, allowing you to direct attention away from pain sensations when appropriate.

Emotional Regulation: Regular mindfulness practice increases activity in brain regions associated with emotional regulation while decreasing reactivity in the amygdala, the brain's alarm center.

Interoceptive Awareness: Mindfulness enhances your ability to accurately perceive internal bodily sensations without automatically interpreting them as threatening.

Default Mode Network Modification: Mindfulness practice reduces activity in the default mode network, brain regions associated with rumination and self-referential thinking that often amplify pain experiences.

Results indicated that MBPM had enhancing effects on cognitive performance related to attention, inhibitory control, and psychological well-being. Results also indicated several significant relationships between emotion regulation, pain severity, pain interference, interoception, and cognitive performance. Interoception may play a key role in improving cognitive and emotion processing function in chronic pain patients exposed to mindfulness.

Cognitive Functional Therapy

Cognitive Functional Therapy (CFT) combines pain neuroscience education with movement retraining and cognitive interventions. CFT specifically targets the multidimensional nature of chronic pain by addressing cognitive, emotional, physical, and behavioral factors simultaneously.

The core components of CFT include:

Cognitive Targeting: Identifying and modifying unhelpful beliefs about pain, movement, and the body that contribute to central sensitization.

Functional Movement Training: Gradual exposure to movements and activities in a graded manner that promotes normal movement patterns while reducing protective behaviors.

Lifestyle Modification: Addressing sleep, stress, and activity patterns that influence pain processing.

Behavioral Experiments: Testing catastrophic predictions about movement and activity to provide corrective experiences that update pain-related beliefs.

Transcranial Stimulation: Direct Brain Modulation

Recent advances in non-invasive brain stimulation represent some of the most exciting developments in pain neuroscience. The authors examined various noninvasive methods, such as transcranial magnetic stimulation, transcranial direct current stimulation and ultrasound, which target specific brain areas involved in pain processing. These techniques can alter neural activity without surgery, offering a safer alternative to traditional treatments.

Transcranial Magnetic Stimulation (TMS)

TMS uses focused magnetic pulses to modulate activity in specific brain regions associated with pain processing. The findings suggest that these methods can reduce pain by influencing neural circuits and promoting beneficial changes in the brain. However, the effects are often temporary, highlighting the need for further research to develop long-lasting solutions.

High-frequency TMS applied to the motor cortex has shown particular promise for chronic neuropathic pain conditions. The mechanism appears to involve:

Motor Cortex Modulation: Stimulation of the primary motor cortex influences descending pain inhibitory pathways, reducing pain signal transmission in the spinal cord.

Neuroplasticity Induction: Repeated TMS sessions promote long-term potentiation in pain-inhibiting neural circuits while reducing activity in pain-facilitating pathways.

Network Effects: TMS influences entire brain networks rather than just the stimulated region, creating widespread changes in pain processing circuits.

Transcranial Direct Current Stimulation (tDCS)

tDCS applies weak electrical currents to specific brain regions to modulate neuronal excitability. Unlike TMS, which uses magnetic pulses, tDCS provides sustained modulation of brain activity during and after stimulation sessions.

Research demonstrates tDCS effectiveness for various chronic pain conditions:

Fibromyalgia: Studies show that anodal tDCS applied to the motor cortex can significantly reduce pain intensity and improve quality of life in fibromyalgia patients.

Chronic Low Back Pain: tDCS combined with other interventions shows enhanced effectiveness compared to single-modality treatments.

Neuropathic Pain: Multiple studies demonstrate tDCS's ability to reduce neuropathic pain intensity and improve functional outcomes.

Focused Ultrasound

Focused ultrasound represents the newest frontier in non-invasive brain stimulation for pain. Kim, H.-J. et al. Long-lasting forms of plasticity through patterned ultrasound-induced brainwave entrainment. di Biase, L. et al. Focused ultrasound (FUS) for chronic pain management: approved and potential applications.

This technology offers several advantages over other stimulation methods:

Precision: Ultrasound can target deep brain structures with millimeter precision without affecting surrounding tissues.

Depth: Unlike TMS and tDCS, focused ultrasound can reach deep brain regions involved in pain processing.

Real-time Guidance: MRI guidance allows for precise targeting and real-time monitoring of treatment effects.

Creating New Neural Pathways

The ultimate goal of neuroplasticity-based interventions is creating new neural pathways that bypass or override maladaptive pain circuits. This process involves several complementary mechanisms:

Synaptic Strengthening in Inhibitory Pathways

The brain contains extensive pain inhibitory systems that naturally suppress pain signals. In chronic pain conditions, these inhibitory systems often become weakened or dysfunctional. Neuroplasticity training can systematically strengthen these pathways through:

Repeated Activation: Consistently engaging pain inhibitory systems through specific mental practices strengthens synaptic connections in these circuits.

Cognitive Loading: Mental tasks that require attention and cognitive resources activate prefrontal cortex regions that naturally inhibit pain processing.

Positive Emotional States: Cultivating positive emotions activates endogenous opioid and cannabinoid systems that naturally reduce pain.

Structural Brain Changes

Advanced neuroimaging studies reveal that sustained neuroplasticity training produces measurable structural changes in the brain:

Gray Matter Increases: Studies show increased gray matter volume in brain regions associated with pain modulation, attention control, and emotional regulation.

White Matter Integrity: Improved connectivity between brain regions through enhanced white matter tract integrity.

Cortical Thickness: Increased cortical thickness in areas involved in sensory processing and cognitive control.

Functional Network Reorganization

Neuroplasticity training promotes beneficial changes in how different brain networks communicate:

Salience Network Normalization: Reduced hyperactivity in the salience network, which inappropriately flags neutral sensations as threatening in chronic pain.

Default Mode Network Regulation: Decreased rumination and pain-focused attention through default mode network modification.

Executive Control Enhancement: Strengthened executive control networks that can override automatic pain responses.

Integration and Optimization Strategies

Maximizing neuroplasticity-based healing requires strategic integration of multiple approaches:

Sequential Protocol Development

Research suggests optimal sequencing of interventions:

1. **Foundation Phase**: Pain neuroscience education to establish understanding and reduce fear

2. **Activation Phase**: Introduction of mindfulness and cognitive training to begin neuroplastic changes

3. **Integration Phase**: Combination of brain stimulation with behavioral interventions for enhanced effectiveness

4. **Maintenance Phase**: Sustained practice to consolidate neuroplastic changes

Personalization Based on Neural Profiles

Emerging research suggests that individual differences in brain structure and function influence treatment response. Future approaches will likely incorporate:

Neuroimaging-Guided Treatment: Using brain scans to identify optimal stimulation targets and treatment approaches.

Biomarker-Informed Protocols: Tailoring interventions based on inflammatory markers, stress hormones, and other biological indicators.

Cognitive Profile Matching: Adapting cognitive training approaches based on individual cognitive strengths and weaknesses.

Technology-Enhanced Delivery

Modern technology enables more effective delivery of neuroplasticity training:

Virtual Reality Integration: Immersive environments that enhance engagement and effectiveness of cognitive training.

Real-Time Neurofeedback: Immediate feedback about brain activity to optimize training sessions.

Mobile Applications: Accessible tools for daily practice and progress monitoring.

The Future of Neural Rewiring

As our understanding of neuroplasticity mechanisms deepens, new possibilities emerge for chronic pain treatment. Recent investigations have explored the therapeutic benefits of immersive VR experiences combined with BCI-driven interventions for conditions such as chronic pain management. Research by Li et al. (2024) implemented a closed-loop BCI system in VR to deliver real-time neurofeedback during pain distraction exercises.

The convergence of brain stimulation, virtual reality, artificial intelligence, and precision medicine promises increasingly effective approaches to rewiring pain pathways. Your brain's capacity for change—the same neuroplasticity that created your chronic pain—represents an unlimited resource for healing that we're only beginning to fully harness.

Understanding these mechanisms empowers you to participate actively in rewiring your own pain pathways. The techniques described in this chapter aren't just theoretical possibilities—they're evidence-based tools you can begin implementing immediately to promote beneficial neuroplastic changes that lead to lasting pain relief.

CHAPTER 3: THE MINDFUL PAIN REVOLUTION

The Scientific Revolution of Consciousness-Based Medicine

For millennia, contemplative traditions have maintained that suffering is optional—that while pain may be inevitable, our relationship with that pain determines whether we suffer. Modern neuroscience has now validated this ancient wisdom with rigorous clinical trials demonstrating that mindfulness-based interventions can be more effective than many conventional treatments for chronic pain conditions.

Mindfulness-Based Pain Management (MBPM) represents a revolutionary approach that addresses chronic pain at its neurobiological roots. Accruing evidence supports the clinical efficacy of mindfulness treatments in reducing chronic pain symptoms. Recent studies show that MBPM participants experienced significant pain reduction, improved quality of life, and enhanced cognitive function compared to control groups receiving standard medical care.

What makes MBPM truly revolutionary is its ability to work with your brain's natural pain processing mechanisms rather than against them. Instead of trying to block or mask pain signals—the approach of most medications—mindfulness training teaches your brain to process pain differently at the most fundamental level. The result is not just temporary relief, but lasting neuroplastic changes that can dramatically reduce or eliminate chronic pain.

Why Mindfulness Outperforms Medication for Many Conditions

The evidence for mindfulness-based interventions in chronic pain management has reached a tipping point where major medical institutions now recommend it as a first-line treatment. The 2017 clinical practice guidelines issued by the American College of Physicians strongly recommended mindfulness-based approaches, including mindfulness-based stress reduction, as initial treatment for patients with chronic low-back pain.

Superior Long-Term Outcomes

Unlike medications that provide temporary symptom relief while potentially causing side effects and dependency, mindfulness training creates lasting changes in brain structure and function. MBPM had enhancing effects on cognitive performance related to attention, inhibitory control, and psychological well-being. These effects were not seen in the chronic pain treatment-as-usual matched patient control group.

Clinical trials consistently demonstrate that mindfulness interventions produce benefits that persist long after treatment ends. A 13-week cognitive behavioral therapy program with integrated mindfulness meditation reduced depression, anxiety and pain-catastrophizing compared with the control group. Increased level of mindfulness and acceptance were associated with change in psychological distress.

Addressing Root Causes Rather Than Symptoms

Medications typically target specific neurotransmitter systems or inflammatory pathways, providing symptom relief without addressing the underlying neuroplastic changes that maintain chronic pain. Mindfulness training, by contrast, directly modifies the brain networks responsible for pain processing, attention, and emotional regulation.

Research reveals that mindfulness interventions specifically target the neurobiological mechanisms underlying chronic pain:

Central Sensitization Reversal: Mindfulness practice helps normalize hypersensitive pain processing systems by strengthening inhibitory pathways and reducing inflammatory responses in the central nervous system.

Attention Network Modification: Regular mindfulness training strengthens prefrontal cortex regions responsible for attention control, allowing practitioners to disengage from pain when appropriate and engage with pain skillfully when necessary.

Emotional Regulation Enhancement: Mindfulness increases activity in brain regions associated with emotional regulation while reducing reactivity in the amygdala, breaking the pain-fear-avoidance cycle that maintains chronic pain.

Minimal Risk Profile

While medications for chronic pain often carry significant risks—including addiction potential, cognitive impairment, gastrointestinal problems, and cardiovascular effects—mindfulness training has an exceptionally favorable risk-benefit profile. The most commonly reported "side effects" of mindfulness practice include improved sleep, reduced anxiety, enhanced emotional regulation, and increased overall well-being.

The Loving-Kindness Revolution in Pain Management

One of the most distinctive aspects of MBPM compared to other mindfulness-based interventions is its emphasis on loving-kindness, which is manifested in its stress on bringing kindliness and compassion to all forms of meditative awareness, in its teaching of loving-kindness practices utilizing the imagination, and in its six-stage process progressing from the individual to the interpersonal and collective aspects of human experience.

The Neuroscience of Self-Compassion

Research demonstrates that self-compassion practices produce specific neurobiological changes that directly benefit chronic pain sufferers. Studies investigating the impact of an 8-week Mindfulness-Based Pain Management intervention found preliminary data suggesting that oxytocin may play a larger role in modulating pain experience and pain perception through mindfulness than previously considered.

The loving-kindness approach addresses several critical factors that maintain chronic pain:

Self-Criticism and Pain Amplification: Chronic pain patients often develop harsh, critical relationships with their bodies and their pain. This self-criticism activates stress response systems that amplify pain signals. Loving-kindness practice cultivates a gentle, accepting relationship with bodily sensations that reduces stress-induced pain amplification.

Social Pain and Physical Pain Overlap: Neuroscience research reveals that social pain and physical pain activate overlapping brain networks. Feelings of isolation, shame, and disconnection—common in chronic pain—literally amplify physical pain processing. Loving-kindness practice strengthens neural networks associated with social connection and belonging.

Oxytocin-Mediated Pain Relief: Compassion practices increase oxytocin production, which has direct analgesic effects. Oxytocin modulates pain perception by activating endogenous opioid systems and reducing inflammatory responses.

The Two Arrows Teaching in Practice

The core theoretical basis of MBPM is the distinction between "primary" and "secondary" suffering, as explicated in the Buddha's parable of the two arrows in the Sallatha Sutta. According to this teaching, while primary suffering or the unpleasant physical sensations that "come with being human" are inevitable, secondary suffering, which arises from mental "resistance and aversion", is not.

Primary Suffering: The actual physical sensations of pain—throbbing, burning, aching, stabbing. These sensations, while unpleasant, are manageable when approached with mindful awareness.

Secondary Suffering: The mental and emotional reactions to pain—catastrophic thinking, fear, anger, despair, resistance, self-criticism. This secondary layer often causes more distress than the physical sensations themselves.

MBPM programs train participants in kindly present-moment acceptance of primary suffering, leading to the diminishment or disappearance of secondary suffering. This approach doesn't aim to eliminate pain sensations entirely, but rather to transform your relationship with those sensations so profoundly that they lose their power to cause suffering.

Advanced Breathing Techniques for Immediate Pain Relief

Breath-based interventions represent one of the most accessible and immediately effective tools for pain management. Advanced breathing techniques work through multiple mechanisms to provide both immediate relief and long-term neuroplastic benefits.

The Physiological Foundations of Breath-Based Pain Relief

Your breathing patterns directly influence your nervous system's balance between sympathetic (stress) and parasympathetic (relaxation) activation. Chronic pain typically involves chronic sympathetic nervous system activation, which amplifies pain signals and maintains central sensitization. Specific breathing techniques can rapidly shift your nervous system toward parasympathetic dominance, providing immediate pain relief.

Vagus Nerve Activation: Slow, deep breathing activates the vagus nerve, the longest cranial nerve that connects your brain to major organs throughout your body. Vagus nerve activation triggers the relaxation response, reduces inflammatory markers, and activates natural pain relief systems.

Baroreceptor Stimulation: Controlled breathing patterns stimulate pressure receptors in your cardiovascular system that signal safety to your brain, reducing threat detection and pain amplification.

Oxygenation Optimization: Many chronic pain patients develop shallow, restricted breathing patterns that reduce oxygen delivery to tissues. Proper breathing techniques improve oxygenation, supporting cellular repair and reducing pain-generating metabolic stress.

The 4-7-8 Technique for Acute Pain Relief

This evidence-based breathing pattern rapidly activates parasympathetic nervous system responses:

1. **Exhale completely** through your mouth, making a whoosh sound

2. **Inhale through your nose** for a count of 4

3. **Hold your breath** for a count of 7

4. **Exhale through your mouth** for a count of 8, making the whoosh sound

The extended exhalation phase is crucial—it specifically activates parasympathetic nervous system responses that counteract pain-amplifying stress responses. Research shows that regular practice of this technique produces measurable changes in heart rate variability and stress hormone levels.

Box Breathing for Pain Stability

Box breathing creates nervous system stability and reduces pain variability:

1. **Inhale** for a count of 4

2. **Hold** for a count of 4

3. **Exhale** for a count of 4

4. **Hold empty** for a count of 4

This balanced pattern creates coherent heart rate variability patterns associated with optimal nervous system function and reduced pain sensitivity.

Advanced Breath Modulation Techniques

Coherent Breathing: Breathing at exactly 5 breaths per minute (6-second inhale, 6-second exhale) optimizes heart rate variability and activates the vagus nerve most effectively.

Breath Retention Training: Gradually extending comfortable breath holds increases carbon dioxide tolerance, which enhances oxygen delivery and reduces sympathetic nervous system reactivity.

Temperature-Modified Breathing: Breathing through the nose while visualizing cool air on the inhale and warm air on the exhale can provide immediate pain relief through temperature-sensitive neural pathways.

Building a Daily Mindfulness Practice for Long-Term Freedom

The transformation from chronic pain to freedom requires consistent daily practice that gradually rewires your pain processing systems. Research demonstrates that the most significant benefits occur with regular, sustained practice over months rather than sporadic intensive sessions.

The Minimum Effective Dose

Studies investigating optimal practice duration reveal that significant neuroplastic changes begin with as little as 10-15 minutes of daily practice, but optimal benefits require 20-45 minutes daily. Most mindfulness-based programs (MBSR, MBCT, MBPM) consisted of eight weekly group sessions, each session ranging in length from 1.5 to 2.5 hours, supplemented by daily home practice.

Progressive Training Structure

Week 1-2: Foundation Building

- Basic breath awareness (10-15 minutes daily)
- Body scan practices to develop interoceptive awareness
- Simple loving-kindness phrases during pain episodes

Week 3-4: Attention Training

- Concentrated attention practices (15-20 minutes daily)
- Mindful movement with pain awareness
- Expanded loving-kindness practice

Week 5-6: Integration Phase

- Choice-less awareness practices (20-30 minutes daily)

- Mindful daily activities with pain present

- Compassion practices for difficult emotions

Week 7-8: Autonomy Development

- Self-guided practice sessions (30-45 minutes daily)

- Personalized practice routine development

- Integration of informal mindfulness throughout the day

Informal Practice Integration

While formal sitting practice creates the foundation for neuroplastic change, informal mindfulness practice throughout the day reinforces and integrates these changes:

Mindful Transitions: Using transitions between activities as opportunities for brief mindfulness practices, particularly when pain levels change.

Pain Surfing: Approaching pain waves with curious, accepting awareness rather than resistance, using breath and loving-kindness to surf through intense episodes.

Compassionate Self-Talk: Replacing self-critical thoughts about pain with gentle, understanding inner dialogue based on loving-kindness principles.

Technology-Enhanced Practice

Modern technology offers powerful tools for supporting consistent practice:

Biofeedback Apps: Real-time feedback about heart rate variability, breathing patterns, and stress levels helps optimize practice sessions and track progress.

Virtual Reality Meditation: Immersive environments can enhance focus and engagement, particularly beneficial for people with attention difficulties related to chronic pain.

AI-Powered Personalization: Apps that adapt meditation content based on current pain levels, emotional state, and practice history.

Measuring Progress and Maintaining Motivation

Tracking practice benefits requires attention to multiple domains:

Pain Intensity and Quality: Daily tracking of pain levels, but also noting changes in pain quality, duration, and your relationship to pain sensations.

Functional Improvements: Monitoring increases in activity tolerance, sleep quality, and engagement in meaningful activities.

Psychological Well-being: Tracking mood, anxiety levels, pain catastrophizing, and overall life satisfaction.

Neuroplasticity Markers: Improvements in attention, memory, emotional regulation, and stress resilience that indicate beneficial brain changes.

Overcoming Common Practice Obstacles

Pain Interference with Practice: Using pain sensations themselves as meditation objects rather than obstacles, learning to practice "with" pain rather than despite it.

Inconsistent Motivation: Establishing practice habits tied to existing routines, using accountability partners, and focusing on small, achievable daily goals.

Expectation Management: Understanding that benefits accumulate gradually and non-linearly, with some days showing dramatic improvement and others requiring patient persistence.

The mindfulness revolution in pain management offers something unprecedented in modern medicine: a treatment approach that not only reduces symptoms but actually enhances overall well-being while requiring no external resources beyond your own attention and intention. The loving-kindness approach to chronic pain transforms suffering from an enemy to be defeated into a teacher that can guide you toward greater wisdom, compassion, and freedom.

As you develop your mindfulness practice, remember that every moment of aware, accepting attention to your experience—whether pleasant or unpleasant—is literally rewiring your brain toward greater resilience and freedom. The ancient promise that suffering is optional is now validated by modern neuroscience, and the path to that freedom lies in the cultivation of mindful, compassionate awareness.

CHAPTER 4: THE SLEEP-PAIN CONNECTION

Sleep and pain share one of the most profound bidirectional relationships in human physiology, yet this connection remains dramatically underappreciated in conventional pain treatment. Recent groundbreaking research reveals a startling truth that flips traditional assumptions: emerging evidence suggests that the effect of sleep on pain may be even stronger than the effect of pain on sleep. This discovery represents a paradigm shift with immediate practical implications—optimizing your sleep may be the single most powerful intervention you can implement for pain relief.

Between 67% and 88% of individuals with chronic pain experience sleep disruption and insomnia, while at least 50% of people with insomnia report chronic pain. But the relationship extends far beyond simple correlation. The link between sleep and pain is well documented through experimental, cohort, and longitudinal studies that all demonstrate restricted sleep directly increases pain sensitivity, amplifies existing pain, and predicts the development of new chronic pain conditions.

Poor sleep therefore not only affects general health but has a direct impact on inflammation, pain response, and experience. This revelation transforms sleep from a passive recovery period into an active therapeutic intervention—one that can be precisely optimized to promote healing and reduce pain intensity.

Why Sleep Disruption Amplifies Pain More Than Pain Disrupts Sleep

The traditional view assumed that pain causes sleep problems—that discomfort keeps people awake and disrupts normal sleep patterns. While pain certainly can interfere with sleep, cutting-edge research reveals the reverse relationship is actually stronger and more clinically significant.

The Unidirectional Evidence

Microlongitudinal studies employing deep subjective and objective assessments of pain and sleep support the notion that sleep impairments are a stronger, more reliable predictor of pain than pain is of sleep impairments. In one study of adolescents with chronic pain, daily actigraphy assessments revealed significant associations of total sleep time and wake after sleep onset on next-day pain reports. Pain did not prospectively predict any sleep measure.

Similar effects were observed in adult pain clinic patients with a wide range of chronic pain etiologies and comorbid insomnia. Self-reported sleep quality and actigraphically-measured sleep efficiency reliably predicted next-day pain reports, while pain levels showed weaker predictive relationships with subsequent sleep quality.

Neurobiological Mechanisms of Sleep-Pain Amplification

Sleep deprivation produces specific changes in pain processing systems that directly increase pain sensitivity:

Descending Pain Inhibition Dysfunction: Sleep loss weakens the brain's natural pain suppression systems. The rostral ventromedial medulla, a brainstem region crucial for pain inhibition, shows reduced activity after sleep deprivation, essentially removing your brain's natural pain filter.

Inflammatory System Activation: Poor sleep increases levels of proinflammatory cytokines such as tumor necrosis factor alpha (TNF-α) and interleukin (IL)-6, which play crucial roles in pain pathways affecting sleep architecture and leading to sleep disturbances such as insomnia.

Central Sensitization Enhancement: Sleep disruption directly amplifies central sensitization processes, making your nervous system more reactive to pain signals. This creates a vicious cycle where poor sleep increases pain sensitivity, which further disrupts sleep.

Neurotransmitter Imbalance: Sleep deprivation alters levels of key neurotransmitters involved in pain processing, including serotonin, norepinephrine, and dopamine, all of which influence both pain perception and sleep quality.

The Predictive Power of Sleep

Population-based longitudinal studies consistently demonstrate that sleep impairments reliably predict new incidents and exacerbations of chronic pain. People with insomnia are significantly more likely to develop chronic pain conditions over time, even after controlling for other risk factors. This predictive relationship suggests that sleep optimization may be one of the most effective strategies for preventing chronic pain development.

Cognitive Behavioral Therapy for Insomnia in Pain Patients

CBT-I represents the gold standard treatment for insomnia and has demonstrated particular effectiveness for people with chronic pain. It has been shown that CBT-I is efficacious for the improvement of sleep duration, maintenance of sleep, perceived sleep quality, and pain interference with daily functioning in people with chronic pain.

Core Components of CBT-I for Pain Patients

Sleep Restriction Therapy: Paradoxically, limiting time in bed to match actual sleep time increases sleep efficiency and consolidates sleep. For pain patients, this requires careful implementation since pain levels may fluctuate throughout the day, affecting optimal sleep timing.

Stimulus Control Instructions: The bed becomes strongly associated with sleep rather than pain, worry, or wakefulness. Pain patients learn to leave the bed if unable to sleep within 15-20 minutes, returning only when sleepy.

Cognitive Therapy: Addressing catastrophic thoughts about sleep loss and pain amplification. Pain patients often develop fears that poor sleep will worsen their pain, creating anxiety that further disrupts sleep.

Sleep Hygiene Education: Optimizing environmental and behavioral factors that influence sleep, with special considerations for pain management needs.

Pain-Specific Modifications

CBT-I for chronic pain patients requires adaptations that address the unique challenges of managing both conditions simultaneously:

Pain Flare Protocols: Specific strategies for maintaining sleep schedule consistency during pain flares, including modified comfort positions and abbreviated relaxation techniques.

Medication Timing Optimization: Coordinating pain medications with sleep timing to maximize pain relief during sleep periods without causing rebound insomnia.

Activity Pacing Integration: Balancing daily activity levels to promote sleep drive without triggering pain exacerbations that disrupt sleep.

Sleep Architecture and Pain Processing Across Sleep Stages

Understanding how different sleep stages influence pain processing reveals why sleep quality matters more than just sleep quantity for pain relief.

Non-REM Sleep and Pain Recovery

Stage 1 (Light Sleep): The transition period where pain sensitivity actually increases. Brief awakenings during this stage, common in chronic pain, can trigger pain amplification.

Stage 2 (Stable Sleep): Characterized by sleep spindles and K-complexes that actively inhibit sensory processing, including pain signals. Increased Stage 2 sleep correlates with reduced next-day pain sensitivity.

Stage 3 (Deep Sleep): The most restorative sleep stage for pain recovery. Deep sleep promotes tissue repair, consolidates pain-relieving memories, and optimizes neurotransmitter balance. Growth hormone released during deep sleep supports tissue healing and pain resolution.

REM Sleep and Emotional Pain Processing

REM sleep plays a crucial role in processing the emotional components of pain experiences. During REM sleep, the brain processes pain-related memories and emotions, potentially reducing their emotional impact and breaking pain-fear associations.

Chronic pain patients often show reduced REM sleep, which may contribute to increased emotional reactivity to pain and difficulty adapting to chronic pain conditions.

Sleep Spindle Density and Pain Sensitivity

Recent research reveals that sleep spindles—brief bursts of rhythmic brain wave activity during Stage 2 sleep—directly correlate with pain sensitivity. Higher sleep spindle density predicts lower pain sensitivity the following day, suggesting that interventions that increase sleep spindle production could provide significant pain relief.

Creating the Perfect Sleep Environment for Pain Recovery

Optimizing your sleep environment involves addressing both general sleep hygiene principles and pain-specific considerations.

Temperature Optimization

Core body temperature regulation plays a crucial role in both sleep initiation and pain sensitivity. The optimal bedroom temperature for pain recovery ranges from 65-68°F (18-20°C). For pain patients, temperature regulation may be compromised, requiring additional considerations:

Graduated Temperature Control: Using programmable thermostats to create slight temperature drops that promote sleep onset while maintaining consistent temperatures through the night to prevent pain-triggering temperature fluctuations.

Localized Temperature Therapy: Strategic use of heating pads or cooling devices for specific pain areas while maintaining optimal core temperature for sleep.

Light Environment Management

Light exposure directly influences circadian rhythms, which in turn affect pain sensitivity. Pain patients often benefit from:

Blue Light Filtering: Reducing blue light exposure 2-3 hours before bedtime using blue light filtering glasses or device settings.

Morning Light Therapy: Bright light exposure (10,000 lux) within 30 minutes of waking helps regulate circadian rhythms and can reduce pain sensitivity throughout the day.

Blackout Optimization: Complete darkness during sleep periods, as even small amounts of light can disrupt sleep architecture and increase pain sensitivity.

Acoustic Environment Design

Sound management for pain patients involves balancing the need for quiet sleep with the reality that complete silence may increase attention to pain sensations:

White Noise or Nature Sounds: Consistent background noise can mask sudden sounds that might trigger pain responses while preventing hyper-attention to bodily sensations.

Sound Masking for Tinnitus: Pain patients with concurrent tinnitus benefit from specific sound frequencies that mask ear ringing without disrupting sleep.

Ergonomic Sleep Surface Optimization

The sleep surface significantly impacts both sleep quality and pain levels:

Mattress Selection: Medium-firm mattresses typically provide optimal spinal alignment while allowing pressure point relief. Memory foam toppers can provide additional pressure redistribution for pain-sensitive areas.

Pillow Configuration: Strategic pillow placement to maintain spinal alignment while supporting painful joints. Side sleepers with hip pain benefit from knee pillows, while back sleepers with lower back pain may need lumbar support pillows.

Adjustable Bed Considerations: For severe pain conditions, adjustable beds allow fine-tuning of positioning to minimize pain while maintaining sleep quality.

Circadian Rhythm Optimization

Consistent sleep-wake timing synchronizes your body's internal clock with natural circadian rhythms, optimizing both sleep quality and pain management:

Fixed Wake Time: Maintaining the same wake time every day, including weekends, anchors circadian rhythms and improves sleep efficiency.

Strategic Light Exposure: Bright light exposure in the morning and dim light in the evening help maintain robust circadian rhythms that support both sleep and pain recovery.

Meal Timing: Eating the largest meal earlier in the day and avoiding large meals within 3 hours of bedtime supports both sleep quality and reduces inflammatory responses that can amplify pain.

Technology Integration for Sleep Optimization

Modern technology offers sophisticated tools for optimizing sleep for pain recovery:

Sleep Tracking Devices: Wearable devices that monitor sleep stages, heart rate variability, and movement can help identify optimal sleep patterns and track improvements.

Smart Environment Control: Automated systems that adjust temperature, lighting, and sound based on sleep stage detection to optimize sleep architecture.

Biofeedback Training: Real-time feedback about physiological parameters during sleep preparation can help pain patients learn to induce relaxation states conducive to restorative sleep.

The sleep-pain connection represents one of the most powerful and underutilized therapeutic relationships in chronic pain management. By understanding that sleep quality directly influences pain sensitivity through specific neurobiological mechanisms, you can approach sleep optimization as active pain treatment rather than passive recovery time.

The evidence is clear: improving your sleep will improve your pain. The techniques and strategies outlined in this chapter provide a comprehensive approach to transforming your sleep from a source of frustration into a powerful healing ally in your journey toward pain freedom.

CHAPTER 5: ANTI-INFLAMMATORY LIVING

Every meal you eat sends powerful biochemical signals throughout your body, either promoting healing and pain relief or fueling inflammatory processes that amplify chronic pain. The relationship between nutrition and chronic pain is complex and may involve many underlying mechanisms such as oxidative stress, inflammation, and glucose metabolism. Recent research reveals that nutrition plays an important role in pain management, with healthy eating patterns associated with reduced systemic inflammation, as well as lower risk and severity of chronic non-cancer pain and associated comorbidities.

This isn't alternative medicine or wishful thinking—it's evidence-based nutritional pharmacology. A 2024 study from the University of South Australia demonstrated that adopting a healthy diet can reduce the severity of chronic pain, presenting an easy and accessible way for sufferers to better manage their condition. Importantly, these findings were independent of a person's weight, meaning that despite your body composition, a healthy diet can help reduce chronic pain.

The power of nutritional intervention lies in its ability to address chronic pain at the cellular level, modulating the same inflammatory pathways targeted by medications but without side effects. When implemented systematically, anti-inflammatory nutrition can be more effective than many pharmaceutical approaches for certain pain conditions.

The Inflammatory Cascade: How Foods Become Pain Signals

Chronic pain often involves low-grade systemic inflammation that amplifies pain signals and maintains central sensitization. Your dietary choices directly influence this inflammatory state through multiple mechanisms that either promote healing or perpetuate pain.

Pro-Inflammatory Food Triggers

Ultra-processed and sugar-dense foods and drinks contain very high amounts of energy and negligible amounts of beneficial nutrients. These foods are often high in fat, salt, and sugar, and in the case of beverages, caffeine. These nutrients can have a number of effects including increasing circulating inflammatory markers and oxidation and impacting sleep.

Advanced Glycation End Products (AGEs): Formed when proteins or fats combine with sugars at high temperatures, AGEs accumulate in tissues and trigger inflammatory responses. High-temperature cooking methods like grilling, frying, and roasting of processed foods create particularly high AGE concentrations.

Omega-6 Fatty Acid Excess: While omega-6 fatty acids are essential nutrients, the modern Western diet contains excessive amounts relative to omega-3 fatty acids. This imbalance promotes inflammatory prostaglandin production, directly increasing pain sensitivity.

Refined Sugar Impact: High sugar intake causes rapid spikes in blood glucose and insulin, triggering inflammatory cytokine release. The World Health Organisation (WHO) recommends that adults limit intake of 'free sugar' including table sugar, honey, syrups, and sugar-sweetened beverages to less than 10% of total caloric intake.

Food Additive Reactions: Artificial preservatives, colorings, and flavor enhancers can trigger inflammatory responses in sensitive individuals, particularly those with existing chronic pain conditions.

Anti-Inflammatory Food Medicine

Polyphenol Powerhouses: Polyphenols are compounds found in fruit and vegetables that have antioxidant and anti-inflammatory properties. These plant compounds directly inhibit inflammatory enzymes and reduce oxidative stress that amplifies pain signals.

Omega-3 Fatty Acids: Evidence suggests that 3000mg of omega 3 over a 3-month period helps to reduce pain, especially in rheumatoid arthritis. EPA and DHA omega-3 fatty acids specifically reduce inflammatory cytokine production while promoting resolution of inflammation through specialized pro-resolving mediators.

Fiber and Microbiome Modulation: Fiber is found in fruits, vegetables, and whole grains, which are the main components of plant rich dietary interventions. High-fiber foods promote beneficial gut bacteria that produce short-chain fatty acids, which have direct anti-inflammatory effects and influence pain processing through the gut-brain axis.

Antioxidant Networks: Vitamins C and E, selenium, and other antioxidants work synergistically to neutralize free radicals that contribute to inflammatory pain. These nutrients are most effective when consumed from whole food sources rather than isolated supplements.

Mediterranean Diet vs. Ketogenic Approaches

Two dietary approaches have emerged with particularly strong evidence for chronic pain management, though they work through different mechanisms and suit different individuals.

The Mediterranean Diet Advantage

The Mediterranean diet represents one of the most extensively studied anti-inflammatory eating patterns, with robust evidence for pain reduction across multiple chronic conditions. This approach emphasizes whole foods, healthy fats, and anti-inflammatory compounds that directly target pain-generating pathways.

Core Components: High consumption of olive oil, nuts, fish, vegetables, fruits, legumes, and whole grains, with moderate wine consumption and limited red meat and processed foods.

Inflammatory Marker Reduction: Studies consistently show that Mediterranean diet adherence reduces C-reactive protein, interleukin-6, and tumor necrosis factor-alpha—key inflammatory markers that amplify chronic pain.

Cardiovascular Benefits: Since chronic pain often coexists with cardiovascular conditions, the Mediterranean diet's well-established heart health benefits provide additional therapeutic value.

Practical Sustainability: The diet's emphasis on flavorful, satisfying foods makes long-term adherence more achievable than restrictive approaches.

Ketogenic Diet for Pain Relief

Recent research reveals that ketogenic diets may offer unique advantages for certain chronic pain conditions through mechanisms beyond simple anti-inflammatory effects.

Neurobiological Mechanisms: Ketones serve as alternative brain fuel that may stabilize neural excitability and reduce central sensitization. The implementation of a whole-food diet that restricts ultra-processed foods is a valid pain management tool, however a low-carbohydrate ketogenic diet may have potentially greater pain relief benefits.

Rapid Onset Effects: Some patients experience significant pain reduction within days to weeks of achieving ketosis, faster than typically seen with other dietary approaches.

Weight Loss Benefits: For pain conditions exacerbated by excess weight, the ketogenic diet's effective weight loss properties provide additional therapeutic benefit.

Metabolic Optimization: Ketogenic diets improve insulin sensitivity and reduce glucose variability, which can decrease inflammatory responses that amplify pain.

Comparative Effectiveness Research

A 2024 randomized controlled trial comparing whole-food ketogenic diets to standard whole-food diets in fibromyalgia patients found that both groups reported improved quality of life, but the ketogenic group also demonstrated significant improvements in pain interference, weight, depression, anxiety, and inflammation markers.

The choice between approaches often depends on individual factors:

Mediterranean Diet Optimal For: Individuals with cardiovascular risk factors, those preferring variety and social eating, people with digestive sensitivities, and those seeking sustainable long-term approaches.

Ketogenic Diet Optimal For: Individuals with metabolic dysfunction, those needing rapid results, people with neurological pain conditions, and those who respond well to structured approaches.

Critical Micronutrient Deficiencies in Chronic Pain

Common micronutrient deficiencies in people experiencing pain include Vitamin D, Vitamin B12 and magnesium. These deficiencies may exacerbate pain through multiple mechanisms and correcting them can provide significant relief.

Vitamin D: The Sunshine Hormone

Vitamin D deficiency affects up to 80% of chronic pain patients and directly influences pain processing through multiple mechanisms.

Pain Modulation: Vitamin D receptors exist throughout the nervous system, and adequate levels are necessary for optimal function of pain inhibitory pathways.

Inflammatory Regulation: Vitamin D deficiency increases inflammatory cytokine production while adequate levels promote anti-inflammatory responses.

Muscle Function: Vitamin D is essential for muscle strength and function, and deficiency contributes to muscle fatigue that worsens pain conditions.

Optimal Levels: Research suggests that vitamin D blood levels should be maintained above 30 ng/mL (75 nmol/L) for pain management, often requiring 2000-4000 IU daily supplementation.

B12: Neurological Pain Relief

Vitamin B12 plays a role in neurological processes related to pain, particularly in neuropathic pain conditions.

Myelin Synthesis: B12 is essential for maintaining healthy nerve coverings, and deficiency can worsen neuropathic pain.

Methylation Support: B12 supports methylation processes crucial for neurotransmitter production and nervous system function.

Homocysteine Regulation: B12 deficiency leads to elevated homocysteine, an inflammatory compound that worsens pain sensitivity.

Magnesium: Nature's Muscle Relaxant

Magnesium is associated with muscle spasm, inflammation and neuropathic pain, with deficiency being particularly common in chronic pain patients.

NMDA Receptor Modulation: Magnesium blocks NMDA receptors involved in central sensitization, directly reducing pain amplification.

Muscle Relaxation: Adequate magnesium is essential for proper muscle contraction and relaxation, with deficiency contributing to muscle tension and spasms.

Sleep Quality: Magnesium deficiency worsens sleep quality, which amplifies pain through mechanisms described in previous chapters.

Optimal Forms: Magnesium glycinate and magnesium threonate show superior absorption and neurological benefits compared to magnesium oxide.

Additional Critical Nutrients

Iron: Deficiency causes fatigue that worsens pain tolerance and can contribute to restless leg syndrome that disrupts sleep.

Zinc: Essential for tissue repair and immune function, with deficiency slowing healing and increasing inflammatory responses.

Vitamin C: Required for collagen synthesis and antioxidant protection, with deficiency impairing tissue repair and increasing oxidative stress.

Practical Meal Planning for Sustained Pain Reduction

Implementing anti-inflammatory nutrition requires practical strategies that make healthy eating convenient, affordable, and sustainable long-term.

Weekly Planning Framework

Sunday Preparation: Dedicate 2-3 hours weekly to meal preparation, including washing and cutting vegetables, cooking grains and proteins in bulk, and preparing anti-inflammatory spice blends.

Batch Cooking Strategy: Prepare large quantities of anti-inflammatory base recipes like bone broth, vegetable soups, and grain salads that can be modified throughout the week.

Emergency Options: Keep anti-inflammatory convenience foods available for high-pain days when cooking is difficult.

Anti-Inflammatory Meal Templates

Breakfast Foundation: Combine anti-inflammatory protein (eggs, Greek yogurt, or plant-based protein), omega-3 rich fats (walnuts, chia seeds, ground flaxseed), and antioxidant-rich fruits or vegetables.

Lunch Structure: Build meals around leafy greens, add anti-inflammatory protein, include colorful vegetables, and dress with olive oil-based preparations.

Dinner Framework: Start with non-starchy vegetables covering half the plate, add moderate protein portions, and include anti-inflammatory starches like sweet potatoes or quinoa.

Hydration and Pain Management

Dehydration can increase sensitivity to pain and also have other effects on health outcomes, especially in older populations, such as poor wound healing and constipation. Water is essential for circulation of nutrients and waste elimination both of which can influence healing, and pain.

Optimal Hydration: Aim for 2-3 litres per day by incorporating small frequent drinks between meals and foods with higher water content such as soup, fruit and reduced fat yoghurt.

Anti-Inflammatory Beverages: Green tea, tart cherry juice, and turmeric teas provide additional anti-inflammatory compounds while supporting hydration goals.

Overcoming Implementation Barriers

It is important to consider the barriers or practical implications to adhering to a particular eating pattern. These include: ability and access to shop, prepare and cook food, pain flare-ups, cost, culinary skills, sleep, gastrointestinal symptoms, food intolerances, environment, motivation, and mood.

Pain-Friendly Cooking: Adapt food preparation techniques for physical limitations, using ergonomic tools, pre-cut ingredients, and minimal preparation methods during flare-ups.

Budget Optimization: Focus on affordable anti-inflammatory foods like beans, lentils, frozen vegetables, canned fish, and seasonal produce to make healthy eating economically sustainable.

Social Support: Involve family members in meal planning and preparation to reduce individual burden while improving household nutrition.

As part of a multidisciplinary team, a dietitian can work with the patient and their health care team to develop a sustainable plan that improves pain experiences, other health outcomes, and that can be adhered to over a long period of time.

The transformation from pro-inflammatory to anti-inflammatory eating doesn't happen overnight, but the evidence is clear: dietary changes can provide pain relief comparable to medications while improving overall health. By understanding how specific foods influence inflammatory pathways and implementing practical strategies for sustained dietary change, you harness one of the most powerful and accessible tools for chronic pain management.

CHAPTER 6: MOVEMENT AS MEDICINE

Movement represents both the greatest threat and the greatest promise for people living with chronic pain. The wrong type of movement, performed at the wrong intensity or frequency, can amplify pain signals and reinforce the very neural pathways that maintain chronic pain conditions. Yet the right movement, applied systematically and progressively, can be more effective than medications, injections, or even surgery for many chronic pain conditions.

This paradox exists because movement directly influences the neuroplastic changes that either maintain or resolve chronic pain. When you move in ways that challenge tissues appropriately while respecting current limitations, you send powerful signals to your nervous system that those tissues are safe, strong, and capable. When you avoid movement out of fear or push through pain inappropriately, you reinforce danger signals that amplify central sensitization and maintain chronic pain cycles.

The key lies in understanding that not all movement is created equal. Your nervous system interprets movement through multiple filters including intensity, duration, complexity, emotional context, and your beliefs about what that movement means. A gentle yoga stretch performed with mindful awareness sends entirely different signals than the same stretch performed with fear and tension. This is why the prescription of movement for chronic pain requires the same precision and individualization as any other medical intervention.

The Research Revolution: Yoga vs Physical Therapy vs General Exercise

Recent research has provided unprecedented clarity about which movement approaches work best for different chronic pain conditions. The most significant finding challenges long-held assumptions about exercise prescription for chronic pain.

A landmark 2017 randomized controlled trial comparing yoga, physical therapy, and education for chronic low back pain found that yoga was noninferior to physical therapy for improving moderate to severe nonspecific chronic low back pain in a diverse, predominantly low-income population. Both yoga and physical therapy participants had greater improvement in function and pain than education participants, with improvements maintained at one year follow-up.

The implications extend far beyond back pain. A 2024 systematic review and network meta-analysis of 18 studies involving 1,442 participants found that of the various mind and body practices included in the review, yoga plus hot sand fomentation was the most effective in reducing pain intensity and functional disability, and improving the quality of physical life in patients with chronic non-specific neck pain.

What makes these findings revolutionary is that yoga outperformed or equaled physical therapy despite requiring no specialized equipment, individual supervision, or expensive clinic visits. The effects of yoga were similar to those of exercise, yet yoga provided additional benefits including stress reduction, improved sleep quality, and enhanced psychological well-being that general exercise approaches often lack.

For fibromyalgia, a 2022 meta-analysis of six randomized controlled trials found that compared with control groups, yoga therapy was associated with decreased pain intensity, improved sleep quality, and reduced fatigue. The evidence consistently shows yoga's effectiveness across multiple chronic pain conditions, leading the American College of Physicians to strongly recommend yoga as initial treatment for patients with chronic low-back pain.

Physical therapy maintains advantages in specific scenarios. Individual assessment and treatment allows for precise targeting of movement dysfunctions, manual therapy techniques, and education tailored to specific diagnoses. Physical therapy excels when structural abnormalities require specific corrective approaches or when pain conditions involve complex movement patterns that benefit from expert analysis.

General exercise approaches including aerobic training, strength training, and recreational activities provide benefits primarily through cardiovascular conditioning, mood enhancement, and general fitness improvement. While valuable for overall health, these approaches often lack the specific pain-targeting mechanisms found in yoga and specialized physical therapy.

Understanding and Overcoming Kinesiophobia

Kinesiophobia, or fear of movement, represents one of the most significant barriers to recovery from chronic pain. This fear develops through a logical but ultimately counterproductive process where the nervous system learns to associate movement with danger, leading to progressive avoidance of activities that might actually promote healing.

The cycle begins when initial injury or pain episodes create associations between specific movements and increased pain. Your nervous system, designed to protect you from harm, begins flagging those movements as dangerous. Over time, this protective response expands to include movements that are similar to the originally painful ones, then to movements that might potentially cause similar pain, and eventually to broad categories of physical activity.

Research consistently demonstrates that kinesiophobia predicts poor outcomes in chronic pain more strongly than actual tissue damage or pain intensity. People with high fear of movement show greater disability, slower recovery, and increased risk of developing persistent pain conditions regardless of their underlying physical condition.

Overcoming kinesiophobia requires systematic desensitization combined with education about the true relationship between movement and tissue health. The process begins with understanding that movement, when performed appropriately, promotes healing rather than causing harm. Tissues become stronger and more resilient with appropriate loading, while prolonged inactivity leads to deconditioning that actually increases injury risk.

The graduated exposure approach starts with movements that feel completely safe and progressively advances to more challenging activities. This might begin with gentle range of motion exercises performed in comfortable positions, advance to simple strengthening exercises with light resistance, and eventually progress to functional activities that previously triggered fear responses.

Cognitive restructuring plays an equally important role. This involves identifying and challenging catastrophic thoughts about movement and replacing them with evidence-based understanding of how tissues heal and strengthen with appropriate activity. Instead of thinking "This movement will damage my back," you learn to think "This movement is helping my back become stronger and more resilient."

Mindful movement practices provide an ideal framework for addressing kinesiophobia because they combine physical activity with present-moment awareness that helps you distinguish between discomfort and danger. Yoga, tai chi, and similar practices teach you to move with attention and respect for your body's current capabilities while gradually expanding your comfort zone.

Progressive Loading Protocols for Different Pain Conditions

Effective movement prescription for chronic pain follows specific principles that ensure tissues receive appropriate challenge without triggering protective responses that maintain pain cycles.

For chronic low back pain, research supports a graded approach that begins with gentle mobility exercises, progresses to core stabilization training, and eventually incorporates functional movement patterns. The most effective protocols combine spinal mobilization with strengthening exercises that target deep stabilizing muscles while avoiding positions or movements that trigger protective muscle guarding.

Initial phases focus on establishing pain-free movement patterns through gentle range of motion exercises performed within comfortable limits. This might include knee-to-chest stretches, gentle spinal rotation, and pelvic tilting exercises that help normalize movement patterns without triggering defensive responses.

Progressive loading then introduces core stabilization exercises that strengthen deep spinal muscles while maintaining neutral spine positioning. Research shows that motor control exercises targeting the multifidus, transversus abdominis, and diaphragm provide superior outcomes compared to general strengthening approaches for chronic low back pain.

Advanced phases incorporate functional movement patterns that prepare you for real-world activities. This includes lifting mechanics, rotational movements, and dynamic stability challenges that build confidence in your spine's ability to handle daily demands safely.

Neck pain protocols follow similar principles but require additional attention to posture and ergonomics. Initial interventions focus on reducing forward head posture and restoring normal cervical curve through gentle mobilization and strengthening of deep neck flexors. Progressive loading includes resistance training for neck and shoulder muscles while maintaining proper alignment.

For upper extremity pain conditions including shoulder impingement and tennis elbow, eccentric strengthening protocols show particular effectiveness. These involve controlled lengthening contractions that promote tissue remodeling while gradually increasing load tolerance. The key principle involves starting with very light resistance and progressing slowly to avoid triggering inflammatory responses.

Fibromyalgia and widespread pain conditions require the most careful approach to progressive loading. Research demonstrates that low-intensity aerobic exercise combined with gentle strengthening provides optimal benefits without triggering symptom flares. Pool-based exercises offer ideal environments for movement in fibromyalgia because water provides support while allowing full range of motion.

The progression for fibromyalgia typically begins with 5-10 minutes of gentle movement and very gradually increases duration before increasing intensity. The target heart rate should remain in the lower aerobic range (60-70% of maximum) to avoid triggering post-exertional symptom worsening that can set back progress significantly.

Building Sustainable Exercise Routines

Long-term success in movement-based pain management depends more on consistency than intensity. Research consistently shows that modest amounts of regular exercise provide greater benefits than sporadic intense sessions, particularly for chronic pain conditions.

The foundation of sustainable exercise routines involves identifying activities you genuinely enjoy or can at least tolerate consistently. This might be yoga, walking, swimming, cycling, dancing, or any other form of movement that feels accessible and appealing. The specific activity matters less than your willingness to engage with it regularly over months and years.

Routine structure should accommodate the reality of living with chronic pain, including fluctuating energy levels, unpredictable flare-ups, and varying motivation. The most successful approaches include multiple exercise options at different intensity levels so you can maintain consistency even when your condition fluctuates.

A typical sustainable routine might include three components performed on alternating days or combined based on your preferences and schedule. Gentle mobility work such as yoga or stretching can be performed daily and actually helps on higher pain days. Moderate aerobic activity such as walking or cycling provides cardiovascular benefits and mood enhancement several times per week. Progressive strengthening exercises maintain muscle function and joint stability while building confidence in your body's capabilities.

The "something is better than nothing" principle proves crucial for long-term adherence. On difficult days, even five minutes of gentle movement maintains the habit and provides some benefit. This prevents the all-or-nothing thinking that leads to complete abandonment of exercise routines during challenging periods.

Environmental factors significantly influence exercise adherence. Home-based routines eliminate transportation barriers and allow for privacy that some people prefer when dealing with physical limitations. However, group classes or gym environments provide social support and expert guidance that benefit others. The optimal choice depends on your personality, preferences, and practical circumstances.

Technology can enhance sustainability through fitness apps, online videos, and wearable devices that provide guidance, track progress, and maintain motivation. However, technology should supplement rather than replace the fundamental principle of finding movement you enjoy and can perform consistently regardless of external tools.

The most successful long-term exercise routines evolve gradually based on your changing capabilities, interests, and life circumstances. What begins as gentle stretching might eventually progress to more challenging activities as your confidence and capabilities improve. The key lies in maintaining flexibility and curiosity about movement while respecting your body's current needs and limitations.

Movement truly is medicine for chronic pain, but like any powerful medicine, it must be prescribed appropriately, taken consistently, and adjusted based on your individual response. The research is clear that the right movement approach can provide pain relief equal to or superior to many conventional treatments while improving overall health and quality of life. Your journey toward pain freedom through movement begins with a single step, taken mindfully and with respect for your body's remarkable capacity for healing and adaptation.

CHAPTER 7: THE SOCIAL CURE - HOW RELATIONSHIPS HEAL PAIN

Pain, despite feeling intensely personal and isolating, is fundamentally a social experience. Your brain processes social rejection using the same neural circuits that process physical pain, which means that loneliness doesn't just feel painful—it actually amplifies physical pain through shared neurobiological pathways. Conversely, strong social connections activate natural pain relief systems more powerfully than many medications, releasing oxytocin, endorphins, and other compounds that directly reduce pain perception while promoting healing.

This revelation transforms our understanding of chronic pain treatment. While medical approaches focus on tissues, joints, and individual pathophysiology, mounting evidence reveals that social factors may be equally important in determining who develops chronic pain, who recovers, and who continues to suffer. Social support doesn't just make pain more bearable—it literally changes how your nervous system processes pain signals.

Recent research demonstrates that people with stronger social connections show measurably different pain responses in brain imaging studies. When experiencing painful stimuli while holding a loved one's hand or even looking at their photograph, brain regions associated with pain processing show reduced activity. These effects occur automatically, below the level of conscious awareness, indicating that social connection provides biological pain relief through fundamental neurobiological mechanisms.

The Neurobiology of Social Pain and Physical Pain

Understanding why relationships heal pain requires examining how your brain evolved to process both social and physical threats. From an evolutionary perspective, social exclusion represented a significant survival threat. Humans who maintained strong group connections were more likely to survive and reproduce, while those who were isolated faced increased vulnerability to predators, starvation, and environmental dangers.

Your brain developed overlapping systems to process social and physical pain because both represented genuine threats to survival. The anterior cingulate cortex and anterior insula, brain regions that activate during physical pain, also respond to social rejection, loss of loved ones, and feelings of isolation. This neural overlap explains why we use the same language to describe both experiences—social rejection "hurts," we have "broken hearts," and we feel "wounded" by betrayal.

The implications for chronic pain are profound. When you experience social isolation, whether due to pain-related disability, relationship strain, or healthcare dismissal, your brain interprets this as an additional threat. This social threat activates the same stress systems that amplify physical pain, creating a vicious cycle where pain leads to isolation, which increases pain sensitivity, which leads to further isolation.

Conversely, strong social connections activate the parasympathetic nervous system, reduce inflammatory markers, and stimulate the release of oxytocin, endorphins, and other natural pain-relieving compounds. These effects occur regardless of whether the social support directly addresses your pain condition. Simply feeling connected, understood, and valued by others creates measurable changes in pain processing systems.

Why Isolation Amplifies Pain While Community Heals

Chronic pain naturally creates forces that drive people toward isolation. Physical limitations may prevent participation in previously enjoyed activities. Unpredictable symptoms make social commitments difficult to maintain. Well-meaning but unhelpful comments from others can lead to withdrawal from social situations. Healthcare experiences that leave patients feeling dismissed or misunderstood contribute to a sense of alienation from the medical community.

This isolation creates a cascade of neurobiological changes that amplify pain. Loneliness triggers inflammatory responses similar to those seen in chronic illness, increasing levels of interleukin-6, tumor necrosis factor-alpha, and other inflammatory markers that directly enhance pain sensitivity. Isolated individuals show increased activity in brain regions associated with threat detection and decreased activity in areas responsible for emotion regulation and stress resilience.

Sleep quality deteriorates with social isolation, and as discussed in previous chapters, poor sleep dramatically amplifies pain sensitivity. Isolated individuals often develop irregular sleep schedules, reduced sleep quality, and increased rumination that further disrupts restorative sleep patterns.

Mental health impacts of isolation compound these effects. Depression and anxiety, both more common in socially isolated individuals, share neurobiological pathways with chronic pain. The same neurotransmitter systems affected by depression—serotonin, norepinephrine, and dopamine—also modulate pain perception. Social isolation increases risk for both depression and anxiety while making these conditions more difficult to treat.

Community and social connection reverse these processes through multiple mechanisms. Group activities stimulate oxytocin release, which has direct analgesic effects while reducing inflammatory responses. Shared experiences provide perspective that helps normalize the chronic pain experience and reduce catastrophic thinking. Practical support from others reduces stress while increasing confidence in your ability to manage challenging situations.

Social activities that involve physical movement provide additional benefits beyond the movement itself. Dancing, walking groups, gentle exercise classes, and similar activities combine social connection with therapeutic movement in ways that amplify both benefits. The social context makes movement more enjoyable and sustainable while the shared activity strengthens social bonds.

Communication Strategies for Pain Patients and Families

Chronic pain profoundly affects family relationships, often in ways that inadvertently worsen pain while straining emotional connections. Family members frequently struggle with how to respond helpfully to pain episodes, fluctuating capabilities, and the emotional challenges of chronic illness. Pain patients may find it difficult to communicate their needs clearly while managing their own emotional responses to persistent symptoms.

Effective communication about chronic pain requires understanding that family members often feel helpless, frustrated, and confused about how to provide appropriate support. They may alternate between overprotectiveness that reinforces disability and dismissiveness that feels invalidating. These responses typically arise from genuine care combined with lack of understanding about chronic pain mechanisms.

Pain patients benefit from providing clear, specific information about their condition and needs rather than expecting family members to intuitively understand what helps. This includes explaining the difference between acute and chronic pain, describing how pain levels fluctuate unpredictably, and clarifying the relationship between pain and activity levels. Family members often assume that increased activity means decreased pain, or that pain medication should provide complete relief, leading to unrealistic expectations.

Developing a shared language for discussing pain helps improve communication while reducing emotional reactivity. This might involve using numeric pain scales, distinguishing between "hurt" and "harm," or creating specific terms for different types of pain episodes. The goal is creating clear communication that provides necessary information without making every interaction focused on pain levels.

Boundary setting becomes crucial for maintaining healthy relationships while managing chronic pain. This includes communicating limits around activities, social commitments, and emotional support while also identifying areas where you can contribute meaningfully to family life. Pain patients often struggle with guilt about limitations, leading to either overcommitment that worsens symptoms or complete withdrawal that strains relationships.

Family education about chronic pain can dramatically improve relationship dynamics while providing better support for the pain patient. When family members understand that chronic pain involves central sensitization, that pain levels don't always correlate with tissue damage, and that recovery is possible, they can provide more appropriate support while maintaining realistic expectations.

Conflict resolution skills become particularly important when chronic pain affects family dynamics. Pain-related stress can increase irritability and emotional reactivity while reducing patience and tolerance for normal family tensions. Learning to address conflicts directly but compassionately prevents accumulation of resentment while maintaining emotional connections.

Building Therapeutic Relationships with Healthcare Providers

The therapeutic relationship between pain patients and healthcare providers significantly influences treatment outcomes, yet these relationships often become strained due to the complex nature of chronic pain, limitations of current treatments, and systemic healthcare pressures.

Many pain patients have experienced dismissive, invalidating, or inadequate care that creates lasting mistrust of healthcare providers. Previous experiences where providers suggested pain was "all in your head," failed to take symptoms seriously, or provided ineffective treatments while showing frustration can create trauma that interferes with future healthcare relationships.

Effective therapeutic relationships require mutual respect, clear communication, and shared decision-making about treatment approaches. Pain patients benefit from actively participating in their care by preparing for appointments, asking specific questions, and advocating for their needs while also being realistic about treatment limitations and timelines.

Preparing for healthcare visits involves organizing relevant information including symptom patterns, previous treatments and their effects, current medications and dosages, and specific questions or concerns. Many pain patients find it helpful to keep symptom diaries that track pain levels, activities, sleep quality, and other relevant factors that can inform treatment decisions.

Communication with healthcare providers improves when pain patients provide clear, factual information about their symptoms and functional limitations without minimizing or exaggerating their condition. This includes describing pain characteristics, timing patterns, aggravating and relieving factors, and impacts on daily activities using specific examples rather than vague generalizations.

Advocating for appropriate care sometimes requires persistence while maintaining respectful communication. This might involve requesting referrals to specialists, asking about alternative treatment approaches, or seeking second opinions when current treatments aren't providing adequate relief. Pain patients have the right to adequate pain assessment, evidence-based treatment options, and respectful care regardless of their diagnosis or previous treatment history.

Understanding healthcare provider perspectives can improve communication and outcomes. Providers often feel frustrated by chronic pain cases due to limited treatment options, time constraints, and concerns about opioid prescribing. Acknowledging these challenges while clearly communicating your needs and treatment goals can help create collaborative rather than adversarial relationships.

Working with multidisciplinary teams often provides the most comprehensive care for chronic pain conditions. This might include primary care providers, specialists, physical therapists, psychologists, nutritionists, and other professionals who can address different aspects of chronic pain. Coordinating care between multiple providers requires clear communication and active participation in treatment planning.

Creating Accountability Partnerships for Pain Management

Sustainable pain management requires consistent engagement with evidence-based interventions over months and years, which can be challenging when dealing with fluctuating symptoms, motivation changes, and the inherent difficulties of behavior change. Accountability partnerships provide external support and motivation that significantly improve treatment adherence and outcomes.

Effective accountability partners understand chronic pain challenges while providing consistent, nonjudgmental support for your self-management efforts. This might be a family member, friend, fellow pain patient, or professional support person who can help you maintain consistency with exercise routines, mindfulness practice, sleep hygiene, and other therapeutic activities.

The most effective partnerships involve specific agreements about goals, check-in schedules, and types of support rather than vague commitments to "help each other." This might include exercising together several times per week, sharing daily meditation practice completion, reviewing sleep hygiene habits, or providing encouragement during difficult periods.

Peer support from other chronic pain patients offers unique benefits that professional or family support cannot provide. People who have experienced similar challenges understand the frustration, fear, and hope involved in chronic pain recovery in ways that others cannot. They can provide practical advice based on personal experience while offering emotional support during setbacks.

Support groups, whether in-person or online, create communities of people working toward similar goals while providing accountability through regular participation. Many people find that committing to attend weekly support group meetings helps maintain consistency with other self-management activities while providing social connection that directly benefits pain management.

Technology can enhance accountability partnerships through apps that allow shared goal tracking, regular check-ins, and progress monitoring. Some people benefit from virtual accountability partners through online communities, while others prefer in-person connections that provide more direct social interaction.

Professional accountability through regular appointments with healthcare providers, coaches, or counselors provides structured support while ensuring that your pain management approach remains evidence-based and appropriate for your current condition. This might include regular check-ins with physical therapists, periodic consultations with pain specialists, or ongoing sessions with psychologists who specialize in chronic pain.

The accountability relationship should provide support without creating additional pressure or guilt when you're unable to meet goals due to pain flares or other challenges. Effective partners understand that chronic pain management involves setbacks and fluctuations while maintaining encouraging, long-term perspectives on recovery.

Social connection represents one of the most powerful yet underutilized tools for chronic pain management. The evidence is clear that strong relationships provide biological pain relief while isolation amplifies suffering. By understanding how social factors influence pain processing and actively cultivating supportive relationships, you harness your brain's natural healing mechanisms while building resilience for long-term recovery. The path to pain freedom is not a solitary journey—it unfolds through connection, community, and the fundamental human capacity for healing through relationship.

CHAPTER 8: STRESS, EMOTIONS, AND PAIN

Stress and chronic pain exist in a complex dance that can either promote healing or perpetuate suffering. Your internal emotional environment directly influences pain processing through neurobiological pathways that can amplify mild discomfort into debilitating pain or transform severe symptoms into manageable sensations. Understanding and mastering these psychological mechanisms provides some of the most powerful tools available for chronic pain recovery.

The relationship between stress and pain involves far more than simple cause and effect. Chronic stress literally rewires your nervous system to become hypersensitive to threat, including pain signals. Meanwhile, chronic pain creates ongoing stress that further amplifies pain sensitivity, creating self-perpetuating cycles that can maintain suffering long after initial tissue damage has healed.

Recent neuroscience research reveals that stress and pain share overlapping brain circuits, neurotransmitter systems, and inflammatory pathways. The same brain regions that process emotional stress also modulate pain perception. The hypothalamic-pituitary-adrenal axis that governs stress responses directly influences pain sensitivity through cortisol and other stress hormones. Understanding these connections allows you to interrupt pain amplification cycles by addressing their psychological and emotional roots.

The Stress-Pain Amplification Cycle

Chronic stress fundamentally alters how your nervous system processes sensory information, creating heightened sensitivity to all potentially threatening stimuli including pain signals. This occurs through multiple interconnected mechanisms that compound each other over time.

Elevated cortisol levels from chronic stress increase inflammatory responses throughout your body while reducing your natural pain inhibition systems. Stress depletes neurotransmitters including serotonin, norepinephrine, and GABA that normally help regulate pain perception and emotional responses. Sleep disruption from stress further amplifies pain sensitivity through mechanisms discussed in previous chapters.

The cycle typically begins when initial pain or injury creates natural stress responses as your body attempts to protect itself from perceived threat. If this stress becomes chronic due to persistent pain, fear about the future, financial concerns, relationship strain, or other factors, your nervous system remains in a heightened state of alert that amplifies all sensory input including pain signals.

Muscle tension from chronic stress creates additional sources of pain while restricting blood flow to tissues that need oxygen and nutrients for healing. Stress-induced changes in breathing patterns reduce oxygen delivery while increasing muscle tension throughout your body. Digestive disruption from stress affects nutrient absorption and gut bacteria that influence inflammatory responses.

Cognitive changes from chronic stress include increased attention to threatening stimuli, catastrophic thinking patterns, and reduced problem-solving abilities. These mental changes make pain feel more threatening and overwhelming while reducing your confidence in your ability to manage symptoms effectively.

Breaking this cycle requires addressing both the physiological and psychological components simultaneously. Simply treating pain without addressing stress rarely provides lasting relief, while stress management techniques that ignore pain-specific factors often fall short of their potential effectiveness.

Emotional Regulation Strategies That Reduce Pain Intensity

Emotions directly influence pain perception through shared brain circuits and neurotransmitter systems. Learning to recognize, understand, and skillfully respond to emotions provides immediate pain relief while building long-term resilience against pain amplification.

Fear represents the most powerful emotion for amplifying chronic pain. Fear of movement, fear of increased pain, fear of disability, and fear of being dismissed by others all activate threat detection systems that heighten pain sensitivity. These fears often develop logically based on previous experiences but become counterproductive when they prevent engagement in healing activities.

Addressing fear-based pain amplification begins with distinguishing between rational concerns and catastrophic thinking. Rational fear about genuinely dangerous activities serves a protective function, while catastrophic fear about normal activities maintains disability and prevents recovery. Learning to evaluate the actual risk of various activities based on evidence rather than emotion allows for gradual re-engagement with life.

Anger and frustration frequently accompany chronic pain, often focused on healthcare providers who haven't provided adequate relief, family members who don't understand, or yourself for being unable to function normally. While these emotions are natural responses to chronic pain challenges, sustained anger and frustration create stress responses that amplify pain while damaging relationships and reducing treatment effectiveness.

Processing anger constructively involves acknowledging legitimate grievances while channeling emotional energy toward productive action. This might include advocating for better medical care, setting appropriate boundaries with unsupportive people, or engaging in physical activities that provide healthy outlets for intense emotions.

Sadness and grief about losses related to chronic pain deserve acknowledgment and processing rather than suppression or avoidance. Chronic pain often involves genuine losses including physical capabilities, career opportunities, social activities, and future plans. Avoiding grief about these losses can lead to depression that amplifies pain while preventing adaptation to new circumstances.

Healthy grief processing involves allowing yourself to feel sad about losses while gradually investing emotional energy in activities and relationships that remain possible. This process often requires professional support, particularly when grief becomes complicated by guilt, self-blame, or hopelessness.

Anxiety about pain fluctuations, medical appointments, activity participation, and future functioning creates anticipatory stress that often proves more distressing than actual pain episodes. This anxiety frequently involves overestimating the likelihood of negative outcomes while underestimating your ability to cope with challenges.

Anxiety management techniques that prove particularly effective for chronic pain include progressive muscle relaxation, controlled breathing exercises, cognitive restructuring of catastrophic thoughts, and gradual exposure to feared activities. These approaches address both the physical symptoms of anxiety and the thought patterns that maintain anxious responses.

Developing emotional awareness involves learning to notice emotional states as they arise rather than being overwhelmed by them. Many people with chronic pain develop habits of emotional suppression that initially seem protective but ultimately increase both emotional distress and physical pain. Learning to observe emotions with curiosity and compassion allows for more skillful responses.

Trauma-Informed Approaches to Chronic Pain

Growing research reveals strong connections between traumatic experiences and chronic pain development. Adverse childhood experiences, physical or sexual abuse, combat exposure, motor vehicle accidents, and other traumatic events significantly increase risk for developing chronic pain conditions while complicating treatment and recovery.

Trauma affects pain processing through multiple pathways including dysregulation of stress response systems, alterations in immune function, changes in pain perception thresholds, and development of hypervigilance to bodily sensations. Traumatic experiences can create persistent states of nervous system activation that amplify pain sensitivity while reducing natural resilience mechanisms.

Post-traumatic stress disorder frequently co-occurs with chronic pain conditions, creating complex presentations that require specialized treatment approaches. Traditional pain management techniques may prove ineffective or even counterproductive when trauma remains unaddressed. Conversely, trauma treatment that ignores chronic pain may miss crucial factors maintaining both conditions.

Trauma-informed pain treatment recognizes that many chronic pain patients have experienced significant trauma and adapts interventions accordingly. This includes creating safety in therapeutic relationships, providing choices and control over treatment decisions, building on existing strengths and resources, and addressing both trauma and pain simultaneously.

Body-based trauma therapies prove particularly relevant for chronic pain because they address the somatic manifestations of traumatic stress while building positive relationships with physical sensations. Approaches such as somatic experiencing, sensorimotor psychotherapy, and trauma-sensitive yoga help integrate traumatic experiences while reducing pain sensitivity.

Eye Movement Desensitization and Reprocessing therapy has shown effectiveness for both trauma and chronic pain, particularly when pain development followed specific traumatic incidents. This approach helps process traumatic memories while reducing their emotional charge and physical impact.

Recognizing trauma responses in chronic pain treatment includes understanding that certain interventions may trigger traumatic memories or responses. Physical therapy, medical examinations, injections, and other treatments can activate trauma responses in susceptible individuals. Trauma-informed approaches modify these interventions to maximize safety while maintaining therapeutic effectiveness.

Building trauma recovery alongside pain management requires patience and specialized support but offers the possibility of addressing root causes rather than just symptoms. Many people discover that trauma treatment dramatically improves their pain condition while pain management techniques enhance their trauma recovery.

Building Psychological Resilience for Lasting Recovery

Psychological resilience represents the ability to adapt positively to adversity, maintain emotional stability during challenges, and recover effectively from setbacks. For chronic pain, resilience involves developing mental and emotional resources that prevent pain from overwhelming your life while maintaining hope and engagement despite ongoing symptoms.

Resilience building begins with developing a growth mindset about chronic pain recovery. This involves viewing pain management as a learnable skill set rather than a fixed condition, understanding that setbacks are normal parts of recovery rather than signs of failure, and maintaining realistic optimism about improvement possibilities.

Cognitive flexibility allows you to adapt your thinking and behavior based on changing circumstances rather than rigidly applying approaches that no longer serve you effectively. This might involve adjusting activity levels based on daily pain fluctuations, trying new treatment approaches when previous ones plateau, or modifying life goals based on current capabilities while maintaining meaningful direction.

Developing multiple coping strategies prevents over-reliance on any single approach while providing options for different situations and symptoms. Effective coping repertoires include problem-focused strategies for manageable challenges, emotion-focused approaches for situations beyond your control, and meaning-focused methods for maintaining purpose during difficult periods.

Building self-efficacy involves gradually expanding your confidence in your ability to manage pain and maintain meaningful activities despite ongoing symptoms. This develops through successful experiences with pain management techniques, gradual increases in activity tolerance, and recognition of your growing knowledge and skills.

Stress inoculation training helps build resilience by gradually exposing you to manageable stressors while practicing coping skills. This might involve progressively challenging physical activities, difficult emotional situations, or complex problem-solving scenarios that build confidence in your ability to handle future challenges.

Developing psychological resources includes cultivating optimism, gratitude, humor, and other positive emotional states that provide buffers against pain-related distress. These aren't just feel-good approaches but evidence-based interventions that create measurable changes in stress physiology and pain processing.

Meaning-making involves finding purpose and significance in your experiences with chronic pain rather than viewing them as purely negative. This might include helping others with similar challenges, developing empathy and compassion through personal struggle, or discovering inner strength and resilience you didn't know you possessed.

Building support networks provides external resources for managing stress and maintaining perspective during difficult periods. Resilient individuals actively cultivate relationships that provide emotional support, practical assistance, and different perspectives on challenges.

The internal environment of thoughts, emotions, and stress responses provides the context within which all other pain management interventions occur. By mastering these psychological factors, you create optimal conditions for healing while building resources that serve you throughout recovery and beyond. Psychological resilience doesn't eliminate pain but transforms your relationship with it, allowing you to live fully despite ongoing challenges while maximizing your potential for improvement and adaptation.

CHAPTER 9: INTEGRATION PROTOCOL

Creating a personalized pain management approach requires balancing evidence-based interventions with your unique circumstances, preferences, and capabilities. While research provides clear guidance about which approaches work for chronic pain conditions, the optimal combination, timing, and intensity of interventions varies significantly between individuals based on pain type, severity, duration, lifestyle factors, and personal resources.

The integration process transforms isolated techniques into a synergistic system where each intervention enhances the effectiveness of others. Mindfulness practice improves sleep quality, which reduces pain sensitivity and enhances exercise tolerance. Better nutrition supports stress resilience, which amplifies the benefits of psychological interventions. Social connections provide accountability for lifestyle changes while offering emotional support that directly reduces pain intensity.

This chapter provides a systematic framework for creating your personalized pain-free blueprint by assessing your unique pain profile, prioritizing interventions based on evidence and feasibility, sequencing treatments for maximum effectiveness, and establishing sustainable routines that evolve with your progress.

Assessing Your Unique Pain Profile

Effective integration begins with comprehensive assessment of your current pain experience, underlying contributing factors, available resources, and personal preferences. This assessment guides decision-making about which interventions to prioritize and how to sequence them for optimal outcomes.

Pain characteristics significantly influence treatment selection. Neuropathic pain conditions respond particularly well to mindfulness-based interventions and sleep optimization, while inflammatory pain shows stronger responses to nutritional approaches and stress management. Widespread pain conditions like fibromyalgia require gentle, gradual approaches that emphasize nervous system calming, while localized musculoskeletal pain often benefits from more targeted movement interventions.

Duration and severity of your pain condition affects the timeline and intensity of interventions. Recent onset pain often responds more quickly to treatment, while long-standing chronic pain typically requires more comprehensive approaches implemented over longer timeframes. Higher intensity pain may necessitate starting with gentler interventions that provide immediate relief before progressing to more challenging techniques.

Sleep quality assessment reveals crucial information about pain amplification factors. Poor sleep often represents the highest priority intervention target because sleep optimization provides rapid, significant benefits for pain management while enhancing the effectiveness of all other approaches. If you're experiencing significant sleep disruption, addressing this becomes foundational to your recovery plan.

Stress levels and psychological factors influence both treatment selection and implementation strategies. High stress conditions may require prioritizing stress management and emotional regulation techniques before introducing more demanding interventions. History of trauma necessitates trauma-informed approaches that emphasize safety and gradual progression.

Current fitness levels and movement tolerance guide exercise prescription and progression rates. Severely deconditioned individuals need very gradual movement introduction, while those maintaining reasonable fitness levels can progress more quickly to therapeutic exercise intensities.

Social support availability affects implementation strategies and accountability systems. Strong social networks provide resources for maintaining consistency with challenging lifestyle changes, while limited social support requires developing alternative accountability mechanisms and potentially prioritizing interventions that can be implemented independently.

Prioritizing Interventions Based on Evidence and Feasibility

Research provides clear guidance about which interventions offer the strongest evidence for chronic pain management, but practical considerations often determine which approaches you can realistically implement given your current circumstances and resources.

Sleep optimization typically represents the highest priority intervention for most chronic pain conditions due to its powerful effects on pain sensitivity and its foundational role in supporting all other healing processes. Sleep improvements often provide noticeable benefits within days to weeks while requiring minimal financial investment or special equipment.

Mindfulness-based pain management offers the strongest evidence base for psychological pain interventions and can be started immediately without professional supervision. The combination of immediate benefits for stress and emotional regulation with long-term neuroplasticity changes makes mindfulness a high-priority intervention for most people.

Movement interventions require careful prioritization based on your current capabilities and preferences. Yoga shows the strongest evidence for chronic pain conditions and can be adapted for virtually any fitness level, making it an excellent choice for most people. However, individual preferences for group classes versus home practice, gentle versus more vigorous approaches, and spiritual versus purely physical orientations influence optimal selection.

Nutritional approaches provide excellent value for most chronic pain conditions because they address underlying inflammatory processes while supporting overall health. Anti-inflammatory eating patterns can be implemented immediately and often provide noticeable benefits within weeks. The accessibility and safety of nutritional interventions make them high-priority regardless of your current condition severity.

Stress management and emotional regulation techniques become highest priority when psychological factors significantly contribute to pain amplification. If you experience high anxiety, depression, or trauma-related symptoms, addressing these may be prerequisite to benefiting fully from other interventions.

Social support interventions may be essential if isolation significantly contributes to your pain experience, but they often require more time and effort to implement effectively. Building supportive relationships and communication skills provides long-term benefits but may not offer immediate symptom relief.

Professional treatment integration depends on availability, affordability, and your specific needs. Physical therapy, psychological counseling, medical management, and other professional services can dramatically accelerate progress but require balancing costs and time investment against potential benefits.

Timing and Sequencing for Maximum Effectiveness

The sequence and timing of interventions significantly influences their effectiveness and your ability to maintain consistency with multiple approaches simultaneously. Strategic sequencing builds momentum by starting with interventions that provide quick benefits while gradually introducing more challenging techniques as your capabilities and confidence increase.

Foundation phase interventions establish basic practices that support all subsequent efforts. Sleep hygiene improvements and basic stress management techniques provide immediate benefits while creating optimal conditions for implementing more demanding interventions. Pain neuroscience education during this phase reduces fear and builds confidence in your ability to influence your pain experience.

The foundation phase typically lasts two to four weeks and focuses on establishing consistent sleep routines, learning basic mindfulness techniques, implementing anti-inflammatory nutrition principles, and beginning gentle movement within your current tolerance levels. This phase emphasizes building sustainable habits rather than dramatic changes.

Activation phase interventions introduce more structured and intensive approaches as foundational habits become established. This phase typically begins in weeks three to six and includes more formal mindfulness practice, structured exercise programs, comprehensive nutritional changes, and active stress management techniques.

During the activation phase, you begin tracking progress more systematically while adjusting interventions based on your response. This phase often produces the most noticeable improvements as multiple approaches work synergistically while your nervous system begins adapting to healthier patterns.

Integration phase interventions combine all approaches into comprehensive lifestyle changes that become natural parts of your daily routine. This phase typically begins around week eight to twelve and focuses on optimizing the combination and timing of different techniques while building long-term sustainability.

The integration phase emphasizes developing intuitive understanding of what works best for your unique situation while maintaining consistency during challenging periods. You learn to adjust your approach based on changing circumstances while maintaining core practices that support ongoing recovery.

Maintenance phase interventions focus on sustaining improvements while continuing gradual progress toward your long-term goals. This ongoing phase emphasizes flexibility, prevention of setbacks, and continued learning about optimizing your pain management approach.

Creating Sustainable Daily, Weekly, and Monthly Routines

Sustainable pain management requires embedding evidence-based practices into realistic routines that accommodate your current lifestyle while promoting gradual positive changes. Effective routines balance consistency with flexibility, allowing for adaptation to changing circumstances while maintaining therapeutic momentum.

Daily routines provide the foundation for consistent implementation of core interventions. Morning routines might include mindfulness meditation, gentle movement, anti-inflammatory breakfast choices, and stress management techniques that set positive tone for the entire day. These morning practices often prove most sustainable because they occur before daily demands interfere with intentions.

Evening routines support restorative sleep while processing daily stress that might otherwise amplify pain overnight. Evening practices might include progressive muscle relaxation, gratitude journaling, gentle stretching, and sleep hygiene activities that promote deep, restorative sleep.

Throughout the day, micro-practices maintain therapeutic benefits without requiring significant time investment. Brief mindfulness moments during transitions, anti-inflammatory snack choices, posture awareness during work activities, and stress-reducing breathing techniques can be integrated into busy schedules while providing cumulative benefits.

Weekly routines provide structure for more intensive interventions that support daily practices. This might include longer movement sessions, meal preparation for healthy eating, social activities that provide connection and support, and planning sessions that maintain focus on recovery goals.

Weekly check-ins with yourself or accountability partners help maintain motivation while allowing for necessary adjustments to your approach. These sessions provide opportunities to celebrate progress, address challenges, and refine techniques based on your evolving understanding of what works best.

Monthly routines support long-term planning and major adjustments to your pain management approach. Monthly assessments of progress, goal refinement, and intervention modifications ensure that your approach evolves appropriately as your condition improves and your life circumstances change.

Monthly activities might include comprehensive progress reviews, professional appointment scheduling, social activity planning, and learning new techniques that enhance your existing toolkit. These longer-term perspectives prevent discouragement during temporary setbacks while maintaining focus on overall recovery trajectory.

Measuring Progress and Adjusting Your Approach

Effective pain management requires systematic tracking of multiple outcome measures that provide objective feedback about intervention effectiveness while maintaining motivation during gradual improvement processes.

Pain intensity tracking remains important but should be balanced with functional improvement measures that often change before pain levels decrease significantly. Daily pain ratings using zero to ten scales provide baseline information, but tracking should also include pain quality, duration, and your emotional response to pain episodes.

Functional improvement measures often show changes before pain intensity reductions and provide more meaningful indicators of recovery progress. These might include activity tolerance, exercise capacity, sleep quality, emotional regulation, social engagement, and ability to pursue meaningful goals despite ongoing symptoms.

Quality of life indicators capture the broader impacts of your pain management approach beyond simple symptom reduction. Life satisfaction, relationship quality, work performance, recreational activity participation, and overall sense of wellbeing often improve dramatically even when pain persists at noticeable levels.

Intervention adherence tracking helps identify which approaches you're implementing consistently versus those that prove difficult to maintain. This information guides adjustments to make your plan more realistic and sustainable while identifying barriers that need addressing.

Progress tracking should include both objective measures and subjective assessments of your overall trajectory. Objective measures might include sleep tracker data, exercise performance metrics, pain frequency and intensity logs, and standardized questionnaires about function and quality of life.

Subjective assessments capture changes that may not show up in formal measurements but represent meaningful improvements in your daily experience. These might include increased confidence in your ability to manage pain, reduced fear about future functioning, improved relationships, and greater sense of hope about recovery.

Regular progress reviews allow for systematic adjustment of your approach based on accumulated evidence about what works best for your unique situation. These reviews might occur weekly during initial implementation phases and monthly during maintenance phases.

Adjustment strategies should be based on specific patterns rather than day-to-day fluctuations. If sleep interventions aren't providing expected benefits after several weeks of consistent implementation, modifications to your approach or additional professional support may be needed. If mindfulness practice becomes inconsistent, examining barriers and adjusting timing or techniques may restore adherence.

Plateau periods are normal during chronic pain recovery and shouldn't trigger dramatic changes to approaches that have been working. Instead, plateaus often indicate readiness to progress to more challenging interventions or opportunities to deepen existing practices.

Your personalized pain-free blueprint evolves continuously as you implement evidence-based interventions, track their effectiveness, and adjust based on your unique response patterns. The integration process transforms individual techniques into a comprehensive lifestyle approach that addresses all dimensions of chronic pain while remaining sustainable within your real-world circumstances. Success comes not from perfect implementation but from consistent engagement with approaches that science shows can provide genuine relief and lasting recovery.

CHAPTER 10: LIVING BEYOND PAIN

Recovery from chronic pain doesn't end with symptom reduction—it begins with learning to live fully while maintaining the gains you've achieved. This final phase of your journey requires different skills than those needed for initial improvement. Where early recovery focuses on implementing new interventions and managing symptoms, sustained recovery emphasizes maintaining beneficial changes while building resilience against future challenges.

Living beyond pain means developing a new relationship with your body and your capabilities. You learn to trust your body's strength while respecting its signals. You maintain therapeutic practices not from desperation but from self-care. You engage with life's challenges confident in your ability to adapt without losing the progress you've worked so hard to achieve.

This chapter addresses the realities of long-term recovery, including managing inevitable setbacks, building antifragility that makes you stronger through challenges, creating meaning and purpose that transcend your pain experience, and preparing for future advances in pain science that will continue expanding your options for sustained recovery.

Understanding and Managing Pain Flares Without Panic

Pain flares are temporary increases in pain intensity that occur during recovery from chronic pain conditions. Rather than indicating treatment failure or permanent setbacks, flares represent normal aspects of the healing process that become less frequent and less intense as recovery progresses.

Understanding flare patterns helps distinguish between temporary symptom increases and genuine setbacks requiring intervention modifications. Most flares follow predictable patterns related to stress, sleep disruption, activity changes, weather patterns, hormonal fluctuations, or temporary lapses in self-care practices. Recognizing these patterns allows for proactive management rather than reactive panic.

Flare triggers often involve combinations of factors rather than single causes. A period of high work stress combined with poor sleep and reduced exercise might trigger a flare that wouldn't occur with any single factor alone. Weather changes don't directly cause flares but can increase pain sensitivity when combined with other stressors. Understanding these interactions helps you identify and modify contributing factors.

The emotional response to flares significantly influences their intensity and duration. Panic, catastrophic thinking, and fear about permanent worsening amplify pain signals while interfering with effective management strategies. Conversely, approaching flares with calm acceptance and confidence in your management skills reduces their impact while facilitating faster resolution.

Developing a flare management protocol provides structured responses that prevent panic while addressing symptoms effectively. This protocol should include immediate comfort measures, modifications to daily activities, intensification of helpful interventions, and decision points about when to seek additional support.

Immediate comfort measures might include gentle heat or cold application, modified positions that reduce stress on painful areas, breathing exercises for stress management, and gentle movement within tolerable limits. These measures provide symptom relief while maintaining your sense of control and competence.

Activity modification during flares involves reducing intensity without eliminating beneficial activities entirely. This might mean shorter exercise sessions rather than complete rest, simplified meal preparation rather than abandoning anti-inflammatory eating, or brief mindfulness practices rather than skipping meditation entirely. The goal is maintaining therapeutic momentum while respecting current limitations.

Intensifying helpful interventions during flares can accelerate recovery while building confidence in your management abilities. This might include extra sleep, increased mindfulness practice, additional stress management techniques, or temporary dietary modifications that reduce inflammation. These intensified approaches often resolve flares more quickly than passive waiting.

Communication strategies help maintain social support during flares without triggering unhelpful responses from others. Family members and friends often react with worry or unsolicited advice during flares, which can increase your stress while undermining confidence. Preparing clear, calm explanations about flare management helps others provide appropriate support.

Building Antifragility: Becoming Stronger Through Challenges

Antifragility, a concept developed by Nassim Taleb, describes systems that become stronger when exposed to stress and challenges rather than simply surviving them. For chronic pain recovery, antifragility means developing the capacity to use setbacks, challenges, and even pain episodes as opportunities for growth and strengthening rather than experiences that diminish your capabilities.

Building antifragility begins with reframing challenges as growth opportunities rather than threats to your recovery. This doesn't mean welcoming pain or minimizing its impact, but rather approaching difficulties with curiosity about what they might teach you and confidence in your ability to emerge stronger.

Physical antifragility develops through progressive challenges that strengthen your body's capacity to handle stress. This might involve gradually increasing exercise intensity, trying new movement patterns, or engaging in activities that previously seemed impossible. Each successful challenge builds confidence while demonstrating your body's remarkable capacity for adaptation and growth.

Psychological antifragility emerges through successfully navigating emotional challenges while maintaining perspective and hope. This includes managing disappointment when progress stalls, dealing with skepticism from others about your recovery, and maintaining motivation during periods when benefits aren't immediately apparent.

The growth mindset forms the foundation of antifragility by viewing abilities and skills as developable rather than fixed. Instead of thinking "I can't handle stress without increased pain," you learn to think "I'm developing better stress management skills that reduce pain amplification." This shift in perspective transforms challenges into opportunities for skill development.

Stress inoculation builds antifragility by gradually exposing yourself to manageable stressors while practicing coping skills. This might involve progressively challenging social situations, physical activities, or emotional experiences that help you discover your expanding capabilities.

Learning from setbacks rather than being defeated by them represents a crucial aspect of antifragility. Each challenging experience provides information about what works, what doesn't, and what adjustments might improve your outcomes. This learning orientation transforms setbacks into valuable feedback rather than evidence of failure.

Developing redundancy in your pain management approach creates antifragility by ensuring that temporary disruption of one intervention doesn't compromise your entire recovery. If injury prevents your usual exercise routine, you have meditation and nutrition practices that maintain momentum. If stress disrupts sleep, you have movement and social support practices that provide stability.

Building margins of safety involves maintaining practices slightly beyond what seems necessary during good periods so you have reserves during challenging times. This might mean maintaining meditation practice even when pain is minimal, continuing anti-inflammatory eating during periods of reduced symptoms, or preserving social connections even when you feel capable of managing independently.

The Role of Meaning, Purpose, and Identity in Sustained Recovery

Sustainable recovery from chronic pain requires more than symptom management—it demands rebuilding identity, purpose, and meaning that extend beyond your pain experience. Many people find that chronic pain has consumed so much of their identity that recovery requires discovering who they are when pain no longer dominates their existence.

Identity reconstruction involves separating your sense of self from your pain experience while integrating lessons learned during your recovery journey. This process often reveals strengths, resilience, and capabilities you didn't know you possessed while helping you release limiting beliefs about your potential that developed during periods of high symptoms.

The transition from "chronic pain patient" to "person who has experienced chronic pain" represents a crucial shift in self-concept. This doesn't mean denying your experience or minimizing its impact, but rather expanding your identity beyond your medical condition to encompass your full human complexity.

Meaning-making involves finding significance and purpose in your pain experience that transforms suffering into wisdom. Many people discover that their struggles with chronic pain have developed empathy, resilience, and understanding that benefits others facing similar challenges. This meaning doesn't justify the pain but helps integrate the experience into a meaningful life narrative.

Contributing to others who face similar challenges often emerges naturally during recovery and provides powerful sources of meaning and purpose. This might involve formal peer support, sharing your experience through writing or speaking, or simply being a supportive presence for others beginning their recovery journey.

Pursuing previously abandoned goals or discovering new purposes provides forward momentum that sustains motivation during challenging periods. Chronic pain often forces temporary abandonment of important goals, but recovery opens possibilities for resuming meaningful pursuits or discovering entirely new directions.

Career and vocational considerations may require significant adjustments based on your recovery progress and any remaining limitations. Some people return to previous work with accommodations, others discover new career paths that better align with their values and capabilities, and still others find meaning through volunteer work or creative pursuits.

Relationship evolution often accompanies recovery as you develop new ways of connecting with others that aren't centered around your pain experience. Family dynamics shift as you resume more active roles, friendships deepen through shared meaningful activities, and new relationships form around current interests rather than shared suffering.

Spiritual and philosophical growth frequently emerges from the crucible of chronic pain recovery. Many people develop deeper appreciation for life's simple pleasures, greater compassion for others' struggles, and clearer understanding of what matters most. These spiritual dimensions provide stability and perspective that support long-term recovery.

Future-Proofing Your Recovery with Emerging Technologies

The field of pain management continues evolving rapidly with new technologies, treatments, and understanding that will expand your options for sustained recovery. Staying informed about these developments while maintaining core evidence-based practices ensures you can benefit from advances without abandoning approaches that currently serve you well.

Digital therapeutics represent one of the fastest-growing areas in pain management, with smartphone apps, virtual reality programs, and artificial intelligence systems providing increasingly sophisticated support for self-management. These tools often provide personalized guidance, real-time feedback, and accessibility advantages over traditional treatment approaches.

Artificial intelligence applications in pain management include personalized treatment recommendations based on your specific symptom patterns, predictive algorithms that help prevent flares before they occur, and intelligent coaching systems that adapt to your changing needs over time. These technologies augment rather than replace human connection and professional guidance.

Virtual and augmented reality applications for pain management continue expanding beyond research settings into practical tools for home use. These technologies provide immersive environments for movement training, relaxation practice, and exposure therapy for kinesiophobia while offering engaging ways to maintain therapeutic practices.

Wearable technology advances provide increasingly sophisticated monitoring of sleep patterns, stress levels, activity tolerance, and other factors that influence pain experience. Future devices will likely provide real-time biofeedback and personalized recommendations for optimizing your pain management approach based on continuous physiological monitoring.

Telemedicine and remote monitoring capabilities expand access to specialized care while reducing barriers to maintaining professional support during recovery. These technologies enable regular check-ins with healthcare providers, participation in group programs regardless of location, and access to specialists who might not be available locally.

Precision medicine approaches increasingly tailor treatments based on genetic profiles, inflammatory markers, stress response patterns, and other individual characteristics. Future pain management will likely include personalized treatment protocols based on biomarker analysis that predicts which interventions will work best for your unique physiology.

Brain stimulation technologies continue advancing with more precise targeting, improved effectiveness, and enhanced accessibility. Future developments may include home-based devices that provide targeted brain stimulation for pain relief while requiring minimal professional supervision.

Nutritional advances include personalized dietary recommendations based on genetic testing, microbiome analysis, and inflammatory marker assessment. Future nutrition approaches for pain management will likely provide increasingly specific guidance about optimal foods and supplements for your individual needs.

Integration platforms that coordinate multiple technologies and treatment approaches will likely emerge to help manage the complexity of personalized pain management while ensuring that various interventions work synergistically rather than at cross-purposes.

Staying current with emerging developments while maintaining critical evaluation skills ensures you can benefit from legitimate advances without being drawn to unproven treatments that promise unrealistic results. This involves following reputable sources, discussing new options with qualified healthcare providers, and maintaining realistic expectations about novel approaches.

Your journey toward sustained pain freedom continues evolving as both your recovery progresses and new possibilities emerge through scientific advancement. The foundation you've built through evidence-based lifestyle changes, psychological resilience, and strong support networks provides stability for incorporating beneficial innovations while maintaining the progress you've achieved.

Living beyond pain means embracing uncertainty about the future while maintaining confidence in your ability to adapt and thrive regardless of what challenges emerge. You've developed not just pain management skills but life skills that serve you in facing any adversity with resilience, wisdom, and hope. Your pain-free future isn't just about the absence of symptoms—it's about the presence of vitality, purpose, and joy that make life worth living regardless of what tomorrow may bring.

CONCLUSION

You now possess something that didn't exist just decades ago: a comprehensive, evidence-based roadmap to freedom from chronic pain. The ten chapters you've just completed represent the culmination of thousands of research studies, clinical trials, and breakthrough discoveries that have fundamentally transformed our understanding of chronic pain and recovery.

This isn't just another pain management book—it's a blueprint for neurobiological transformation. You've learned that your brain constructs your pain experience through complex networks that can be rewired, that your sleep quality influences pain more powerfully than most medications, that specific foods can reduce inflammation as effectively as drugs, and that mindfulness practices can outperform traditional treatments for many conditions.

Most importantly, you've discovered that chronic pain is not a life sentence but a changeable condition that responds to the right combination of interventions applied consistently over time.

The Paradigm Shift

The old paradigm treated chronic pain as a structural problem requiring structural solutions—stronger medications, more invasive procedures, resigned acceptance of limitations. This approach left millions of people trapped in cycles of suffering, dependence, and progressive disability.

The new paradigm recognizes chronic pain as a learned neurobiological pattern that can be unlearned through targeted interventions that address the whole person. Your pain experience emerges from the complex interaction of neuroplasticity, sleep quality, nutrition, movement, social connections, stress responses, and psychological factors. By addressing these systematically, you influence the very mechanisms that create and maintain chronic pain.

This shift from passive patient to active participant in your healing represents more than a change in treatment approach—it's a reclamation of your personal power over your body's most fundamental protective system.

The Evidence-Based Foundation

Every strategy in this book rests on rigorous scientific evidence. Mindfulness-Based Pain Management shows superior outcomes to traditional treatments in randomized controlled trials. Sleep optimization demonstrates more powerful pain relief than many medications. Anti-inflammatory nutrition provides measurable reductions in pain intensity independent of weight loss. Yoga proves as effective as physical therapy for chronic low back pain while offering additional psychological benefits.

This evidence base continues expanding as researchers worldwide investigate new approaches to chronic pain recovery. The techniques you've learned represent the current state of the art, but they also provide a foundation for incorporating future advances as they emerge.

The Integration Imperative

No single intervention provides complete relief for most chronic pain conditions. The power lies in integration—combining neuroplasticity training with sleep optimization, mindfulness practice with movement therapy, nutritional interventions with stress management. These approaches work synergistically, each enhancing the effectiveness of others while creating comprehensive transformation that addresses all dimensions of chronic pain.

Your personalized integration protocol recognizes that recovery isn't linear or predictable. You'll have good days and challenging days, periods of rapid progress and temporary plateaus. The comprehensive toolkit you've developed provides resources for every situation while maintaining momentum toward your long-term goals.

The Journey Ahead

Your journey toward pain freedom has just begun. The techniques you've learned require consistent practice over months and years to produce their full benefits. Neuroplasticity changes occur gradually as new neural pathways strengthen and maladaptive patterns weaken. Sleep optimization may provide immediate benefits but reaches maximum effectiveness with sustained implementation. Mindfulness practice deepens over time, providing increasing resilience against pain amplification.

This timeline isn't a limitation—it's an opportunity. Each day of practice strengthens your pain management capabilities while building overall health and wellbeing. You're not just eliminating pain; you're developing life skills that serve you in facing any challenge with greater resilience and wisdom.

The Ripple Effects

Your recovery from chronic pain extends far beyond personal symptom relief. Strong social connections, regular exercise, healthy nutrition, effective stress management, and mindfulness practice benefit every aspect of your life while positively influencing everyone around you.

Your journey toward pain freedom can inspire others who feel trapped by their own chronic conditions. Your success demonstrates that recovery is possible while your experience provides guidance for others beginning their own healing journeys.

The Call to Action

Knowledge without action remains powerless. The evidence-based strategies in this book can transform your life, but only if you implement them consistently and systematically. Start with the approaches that resonate most strongly with your current situation and gradually expand your toolkit as you build confidence and capabilities.

Begin today. Choose one technique from this book and commit to practicing it for the next seven days. Track your experience honestly and adjust your approach based on what you learn. Build on small successes rather than attempting dramatic changes that prove unsustainable.

Remember that setbacks are normal parts of recovery, not evidence of failure. Every person who has achieved pain freedom has faced discouraging periods when progress seemed impossible. Your commitment to evidence-based approaches during these challenging times determines your ultimate success.

The Promise Fulfilled

The promise made in this book's introduction was that applying these evidence-based approaches consistently would lead to significant improvement in your pain levels, function, and quality of life. This promise wasn't based on hope but on accumulated evidence from thousands of clinical studies and real-world applications.

That promise extends beyond symptom reduction to comprehensive life transformation. You're reclaiming not just your body but your future—the activities you've missed, the relationships that matter most, the goals that chronic pain put on hold.

Your pain-free future isn't a distant possibility but an immediate reality waiting to unfold through your committed action.

The End of Suffering as We Know It

Chronic pain has been humanity's companion throughout history, limiting potential and diminishing joy for countless generations. But you live at a unique moment when science has finally unlocked the mechanisms underlying chronic pain while developing effective interventions for addressing them.

You represent the first generation with access to truly comprehensive, evidence-based approaches to chronic pain recovery. The suffering that seemed inevitable to previous generations becomes optional when you understand how your brain creates pain and how to systematically influence those processes.

The end of suffering as we know it begins with individuals like you who refuse to accept chronic pain as permanent while committing to the disciplined application of scientific knowledge to their own healing.

Your Legacy

Your recovery from chronic pain becomes part of a larger transformation in how humanity approaches suffering, healing, and human potential. Every person who achieves pain freedom expands our collective understanding of what's possible while paving the way for others to follow.

Your pain-free life serves as evidence that recovery is real, that science works, and that hope is justified. Your journey from suffering to freedom inspires others while contributing to a future where chronic pain becomes increasingly rare and recoverable.

The path you're walking leads not just to personal healing but to a world where fewer people suffer unnecessarily because effective solutions remain unknown or inaccessible.

The Beginning, Not the End

This conclusion marks not the end of your pain management education but the beginning of your recovery journey. The pages you've read provide a foundation for a lifetime of learning, growth, and increasing mastery over your pain experience.

Your brain's capacity for positive change continues throughout your life. The neuroplasticity that may have contributed to your chronic pain represents an unlimited resource for healing that grows stronger with practice and purpose.

As you close this book and begin implementing its teachings, remember that you hold the key to your own pain-free future. The science is clear, the methods are proven, and your brain is ready to learn new patterns that lead to freedom.

Your pain-free life awaits. The only question that remains is: When will you begin?

Welcome to your pain-free future. The journey starts now.

www.ingramcontent.com/pod-product-compliance
Lightning Source LLC
Chambersburg PA
CBHW060511280326
41933CB00014B/2921